How to
Succeed at Interprofessional
Education

How to
Succeed at Interprofessional
Education

How to Succeed at Interprofessional Education

Peter Donnelly MB, BCh, BAO, FRCPysch, BA (Open), FHEA, FAcadMEd, FRCPEdin, MMed

Interim Dean, Wales Postgraduate Deanery, Cardiff University, Cardiff, UK

WILEY Blackwell

This edition first published 2019
© 2019 by John Wiley & Sons Ltd

Registered Offices
John Wiley & Sons, Inc., 111 River Street, Hoboken, NJ 07030, USA
John Wiley & Sons Ltd, The Atrium, Southern Gate, Chichester, West Sussex, PO19 8SQ, UK

Editorial Office
9600 Garsington Road, Oxford, OX4 2DQ, UK

For details of our global editorial offices, customer services, and more information about Wiley products visit us at www.wiley.com.

Wiley also publishes its books in a variety of electronic formats and by print-on-demand. Some content that appears in standard print versions of this book may not be available in other formats.

Library of Congress Cataloging-in-Publication Data

Names: Donnelly, Peter, 1958– author.
Title: How to succeed at interprofessional education / Peter Donnelly.
Description: Hoboken, NJ : Wiley-Blackwell, 2019. | Includes bibliographical
  references and index. |
Identifiers: LCCN 2018044857 (print) | LCCN 2018045694 (ebook) |
  ISBN 9781118558799 (Adobe PDF) | ISBN 9781118558805 (ePub) |
  ISBN 9781118558812 (paperback)
Subjects: | MESH: Education, Medical | Interprofessional Relations | Health
Personnel–education | Attitude of Health Personnel | Professional Practice
Classification: LCC R737 (ebook) | LCC R737 (print) | NLM W 18 | DDC 610.71/1–dc23
LC record available at https://lccn.loc.gov/2018044857

Cover Design: Wiley
Cover Image: © Green Flame/Shutterstock

Set in 9.5/12pt Minion by SPi Global, Pondicherry, India

Printed in Singapore by C.O.S. Printers Pte Ltd

10 9 8 7 6 5 4 3 2 1

Contents

Contents

Acknowledgements

I would like to thanks all colleagues, in the NHS and the Wales Deanery, who have helped shape this book. I would also like to thank Katie for her support and patience.

Chapter 1 **Introduction**

The term interprofessional education (IPE) has evolved and developed over a number of decades from as far back as the 1960s. In today's health-service environment across the world enhanced collaborative working across all professionals and disciplines is essential to patient safety and high quality services.

What is this book about? This book is a basic introduction to IPE. The term is being used in the broadest sense and is relevant to learners and teachers across a range of professional settings.

Who is this book for? This book is aimed at:

- learners and teachers across all health fields and other professionals who are new to IPE
- those currently studying on an IPE-focused course or programme
- those currently using IPE to some extent and who wish to enhance their understanding and be signposted to examples from outside their own field

Although the focus of the book is on IPE in health care settings, the principles explored are equally relevant for all sectors. The term 'teachers' is a generic term used to include undergraduate tutors, lecturers and postgraduate educational clinical supervisors and all academic teaching staff. For the purposes of the book no clear distinction has been made between education and training.

Overview of the Book

The book explores the historical background to the development of IPE and brings together evidence of its effectiveness and explores the definitions of a wide a range of terms in relation to IPE. The design principles to support IPE are described as well as examples of IPE in action at organisational levels.

How to Succeed at Interprofessional Education, First Edition. Peter Donnelly.
© 2019 John Wiley & Sons Ltd. Published 2019 by John Wiley & Sons Ltd.

Some of the challenges to the delivery of IPE are highlighted and strategies are suggested for learners, teachers and institutions to maximise the use of IPE. In addition assessment strategies in relation to IPE are explored followed by reflections on the future direction of this important area.

Background

In today's health and social care systems no one clinician can or should work in isolation. The idea that health professionals should learn together so that they can work together is not a new concept, with work published on the subject as far back as the late 1960s (Szasz 1969). At that time there were a number of individual initiatives launched in the UK mainly work and practice based that highlighted the issue of professionals and disciplines working closely together to improve services to patients.

It is often stated that IPE was born formally in the late 1980s following the publication by the World Health Organisation (WHO) of a report into multiprofessional education (WHO 1988). At that time the WHO stated that if health professionals learned together and learned to collaborate as a team early in their career they were more likely to work together effectively in the clinical setting.

Regulators across professions and countries have as a common theme the requirement to work effectively with all colleagues to optimise service provision. *Tomorrows Doctors* (General Medical Council 2009) highlights the importance of respecting colleagues and learning effectively within multidisciplinary teams. This approach is echoed across the professions (General Social Care Council 2010; Nursing and Midwifery Council 2010).

A number of government reports have highlighted the importance of what we now refer to as IPE (Calman 1998; Department of Health 1999).

In the UK it was, however, the NHS Plan (Department of Health 2000) that focused policy in particular on IPE as pivotal to enhancing clinical services for patients. The plan described the introduction of a core curriculum for all NHS staff, more flexibility in career pathways and opportunities for some professions to extend their traditional roles and responsibilities with the needs of the patient at the centre of these reforms/policies.

There have also been a number of high-profile cases that have highlighted the need for effective collaborative working between and across professionals within health and between health, police, social care, probation and the third sector to ensure delivery of safe care; not just health care to the general population (Department of Health 2003; The Joint Commission 2008).

A common theme with these high-profile cases is that poor team working had a significant negative impact on patients. The professional isolation and isolationist mentality and associated behaviour described in some of these cases is perpetuated in part by the way in which each profession trains and learns, from pre-qualifying and post-qualification and then into the workplace. Partnership working is important not just between clinical professions but also between clinical and non-clinical senior management (Francis 2013).

The groundswell of interest in IPE has led to the development of interest groups. On a global scale the World Coordinating Committee All Together Better Health (WCC-ATBH) is a collaboration of worldwide organisations with a focus on the promotion of IPE (see Chapter 5 for more detail). In the UK, the IPE agenda has been facilitated by the Centre for the Advancement of Interprofessional Education (CAIPE). This membership organisation was established in 1987 with the stated purpose:

> *To promote health and wellbeing and to improve the health and social care of the public by advancing interprofessional education (CAIPE website, accessed 30 June 2018).*

CAIPE has published seminal papers including Interprofessional Education Guidelines (Barr et al. 2017).

Challenges

Despite regulators and government policy calling for all professions to work as a team, the majority of undergraduate (UG) and postgraduate (PG) health-related curricula continue to have an emphasis on singular uniprofessional learning, in general in isolation from other professions. This is despite the fact that once these clinicians are in clinical practice they are all required to work in a collaborative partnership. There are a number of reasons for this including confusion in regard to terminology. There is also the issue of a disjoint between UG and PG curricula and a similar disjoint between these curricula and the demands and requirements of the health work place.

A key question is ... is inter-professional learning effective? Is it worth making significant changes to curricula and changes to delivery of the traditional pattern of continuous professional development (CPD)?

The evidence that will be explored in this book is that better team working leads to a better service for patients. This begs the question: Shouldn't inter-professional learning be embedded in every UG and PG programme teaching health work and other related professional work, and on CPD training?

There are various constraints to the introduction of wide spread IPE, including barriers between the separate professions and barriers between disciplines within the one profession. This book will hopefully act as a useful resource for teachers and learners across all health-related professions as an introduction to the principles and practice of IPE. The key message is that partnership working is central to high quality health care for patients and the ultimate outcome for IPE is to enhance professional practice in order to improve the quality of care to those patients.

References

Barr, H., Ford, J., Gray, R. et al. (2017). *Interprofessional Education Guidelines 2017*. Fareham: Centre for the Advancement of Interprofessional Education.

Calman, K. (1998). *A review of continuing professional development in general practice: A report of the Chief Medical Officer*. London: Department of Health.

Department of Health (1999). *Working Together-Learning Together: A Framework for Lifelong Learning for the NHS*. London: Department of Health.

Department of Health (2000). *The NHS Plan. A Plan for Investment, a Plan for Reform*. London: The Stationery Office.

Department of Health (2003). *The Laming Report. The Victoria Clumbié Inquiry – Report of an Inquiry by Lord Laming*. London: The Stationery Office.

Francis, R. (2013). *Report of the Mid Staffordshire NHS Foundation Trust. Public Inquiry*. London: The Stationery Office.

General Medical Council (2009). *Tomorrows Doctors*. Manchester: General Medical Council.

General Social Care Council (2010). *Codes of Practice for Social Workers*. London: General Social Care Council.

Nursing and Midwifery Council (2010). *Standards for Pre-registration Nursing Education*. London: Nursing and Midwifery Council.

Szasz, G. (1969). Interprofessional education in the health sciences. *Millbank Memorial Fund Quarterly* 47: 449–475.

The Joint Commission (2008). *Sentinel Event Alert: preventing infant death and injury during delivery*. 39: April 11. Washington, DC: The Joint Commission.

World Health Organisation (1988). Learning Together to Work Together for health. Report of a WHO Study Group on the Multiprofessional Education of health personnel: the team approach, Technical Report Series 769, Geneva: World Health Organisation.

Chapter 2 Interprofessional Education – The Definitions

Introduction

Interprofessional education (IPE) is not an end in itself. IPE is a learning process or framework to ensure that different health professionals work together effectively to meet the health needs of patients. The IPE movement began in the 1960s with a key driver being the recognition that health professionals do not and should not work in isolation.

The potential advantages of an IPE approach has gained acceptance in a range of different fields. In the field of police work and as a specific example, in the area of child protection, there is a recognition of the need for IPE. The public enquiry into the tragic death of Victoria Climbié (Laming 2003) recommended amongst a range of actions that all child protection officers should receive training in order to help develop the skills and confidence required to challenge the views of other professionals such as consultant paediatricians. IPE is clearly an approach that would enable this inter-professional understanding to be enhanced.

In another sector, the importance of the interaction between housing and health is well recognised. There are complex and diverse relation-ships between the quality of housing, socio-economic status and the health status of the population. In the area of the homelessness, a review by Carlton et al. (2003) highlighted that agencies providing services to the homeless did not communicate well, had competing aims, different cultures and a lack of understanding of the way in which the other relevant agencies worked. It could be argued that IPE would be a method to improve these areas of concern.

How to Succeed at Interprofessional Education, First Edition. Peter Donnelly.
© 2019 John Wiley & Sons Ltd. Published 2019 by John Wiley & Sons Ltd.

Regulatory Background

Health regulators in the United Kingdom (UK) have explicitly included the concept of interprofessional/partnership working in their professional standards.

For example, the General Pharmacy Council (GPhC) states in the standards for pharmacy professionals (GPhC 2017) as of 30 June 2018.

> *Standard 2: Pharmacy professionals must work in partnership with others*
> *People receive safe and effective care when pharmacy professionals:*
> - *work with the person receiving care*
> - *identify and work with the individuals and teams who are involved in the person's care*
> - *contact, involve and work with the relevant local and national organisations*
> - *demonstrate effective team working*
> - *adapt their communication to bring about effective partnership working*
> - *take action to safeguard people, particularly children and vulnerable adults*
> - *make and use records of the care provided*
> - *work with others to make sure there is continuity of care for the person concerned*

The Nursing and Midwifery Council (NMC) within *The Code: Professional standards of practice and behaviour for nurses and midwives* (NMC 2015), under the guidance document *Enabling professionalism* states as of 30 June 2018.

> *'Maintaining professionalism*
> *Registered nurses and midwives practising at graduate level are prepared with the behaviours, knowledge and skills required to provide safe, effective, person-centred care and services. They are professionally socialised to practise in a compassionate, inter-professional and collaborative manner. This is recognised through continuing a registered nurse or midwife status with the NMC. Practice and behaviour are underpinned by the Code and demonstrated through a number of attributes or prerequisites of nursing and midwifery practice...'*
>
> *Enables positive inter-professional collaboration through:*
> - *Partnership approaches to team working*
> - *Clear lines of accountability*
> - *Inter-professional learning/team working opportunities'*

So, there is clear recognition today from all health and social care regulators of the importance of an interprofessional approach to the delivery of a safe and effective service for the population.

There has been a natural evolution of the concept of IPE but it is still argued that there is a lack of clarity in regard to definitions and as a result significant development of IPE has been hindered (Barr 2002). IPE has also been criticised as being merely another 'trend' in medical education, driven by social influences as opposed to sound educational principles and theory (Campbell and Johnson 1999).

Definitions of Key Terms

This chapter provides a brief history of IPE and offers definitions of some key terms. There is a significant overlap between educational strategies in a higher education environment and practice-based initiatives. Also included in this chapter are the definitions of a number of generic educational, health and social care terms that are particularly relevant for IPE and as such have been included for completeness.

The terms discussed in this chapter are often used interchangeably and inconsistently leading to confusion amongst teachers, faculty, learners, organisations and policy developers (Barr et al. 2005). To understand where IPE is at this point in time, it is important to understand the historical context and the evolution and chronology of terms.

Professionalism

Before considering the various terms that are more specific to IPE it is useful to reflect initially on the concept of professionalism itself. In early history, occupations began to evolve and move into what we would now consider a profession. The key milestones marking this transition include fulltime occupation, establishment of training and university schools, codes of ethics and regulation and licencing legislation. The three original professions of law, the clergy and medicine arose through the mediaeval universities in Europe. By the turn of the nineteenth century, with occupational specialisation, different bodies claimed and achieved professional status, including nursing and teaching.

Professionalism has been defined as:

A philosophy, a behavioural disposition, and a skill set that results from one of the fundamental relationships in human interaction.

(Emanuel 2004)

As one example, the concept of *medical professionalism* probably dates back to the late mediaeval times when doctors organised a professional guild

(Sox 2007). Medical professionalism was seen as the art of practicing medicine to a certain set of standards that were regulated by the profession itself. The term as it has evolved has responded to societal and political changes. The key elements it could be argued include a set of behaviours underpinned by values and attitudes. In early society the professions addressed a range of societal issues and in return society afforded these professions:

1 Monopoly status,
2 The authority to decide who could enter the profession, and
3 Influence on government in monitoring their practice.

In essence, there was an implied social contract (Cruess et al. 1999) where there was an acceptance of the balance between altruism and self-regulation.

Although early definitions of the medical profession have been doctor-centred there has been a shift, recognised by regulatory bodies towards a position of medical professionalism as being a social construct, a social contract between doctors and society (Cruess and Cruess 2008).

In the UK, a Kings Fund report (Rosen and Dewar 2004) in exploring the definition of professionalism in today's social structure recommended that the medical profession had to adapt and change, doing more to ensure patient interests are at the centre of their practice.

The public inquiry into Mid Staffordshire (Francis 2013) made a total of 290 specific recommendations. The theme throughout the report is the need for all clinical staff to be professional and genuinely put the patient at the centre of the service.

The origins of professional nursing began with Florence Nightingale, following her experiences in the Crimean war, where she arrived in 1854. She opened the very first school of nursing in London in 1860 and this acted as the catalyst for more schools to flourish allowing those pursuing this profession to be trained in the field. In the UK the General Nursing Council for England and Wales was established in 1919, reorganised as the UK Central Council for Nursing and Midwifery and Health Visiting in 1983 and subsequently formed as the Nursing and Midwifery Council, established in 2002. The purpose of the NMC is to regulate nurses and midwifes in the UK and to protect the public.

Other approaches to professionalism take a broader view. The Humanistic approach places integrity, respect and compassion as central to being key drivers for professionalism. Respect for others is the central element of humanism and Cohen (2007) considers humanism to be the passion that animates professionalism.

In the last 30 years there has been significant societal change including increased knowledge, instant access to knowledge and an increasing consumerist ethos in society. In addition, there have been a number of high profile cases such as Shipman (Smith 2004) all leading to a change in society's expectations of doctors and all healthcare professionals in general.

Proto-Professionalism

Hilton and Slotnick (2005) use the term *Proto-professionalism* to describe the period of time that medical students and trainees doctors go through to develop the state of professionalism. They argue that to develop into the mature professional who displays practical wisdom (phronesis) the medical student requires time to develop the skills, knowledge and experience to acquire professionalism. The question remains … when does for example a medical student become a professional? Is it when they graduate? Or when they start day one in paid employment as a doctor?

Community Care (Care in the Community)

A term often used alongside professionalism and/or team work is *Community Care* (also known as *care in the community*). In simple terms, this is a policy position underpinned by the principle of caring for patients in their own homes rather than in an institution. This concept has been around since the 1950s and was brought under the political spotlight with Enoch Powell's famous 'Watertowers over the Horizon' speech in 1961. Despite widespread criticism of this policy it was in 1983 that the then Conservative government moved the agenda on after the Audit Commission report (Audit Commission 1986).

Why is this clinical model associated with IPE? In essence the entire thrust of Community Care was and still is, of professionals working together to enable individuals with disability, mental health and chronic conditions to live in the community, that is, improved partnership working across professions for the benefit of patients.

Partnership (Partnership Working)

As with many of the terms discussed here *partnership* or *partnership working* has a number of definitions. Although describing the term as a 'slippery concept' the Audit Commission (1998) described it as a joint working arrangement where the individual partners/parties:
1 are independent bodies;
2 agree to cooperate to achieve a common goal;
3 create new processes outside their current organisation to achieve this aim;
4 work to a jointly agreed programme of work;
5 agree to share relevant information/knowledge; and
6 agree to share risks and rewards.

The essence or distinguishing single feature of partnership working is the voluntary as opposed to a contractual arrangement (Powell and Gleddinning 2002).

Uniprofessional Education (UPE)

Uniprofessional education (UPE) is when students or workers from one profession learn together. With UPE in general, the focus is on the mastery of a specific body of knowledge, types of skills and modes of conduct.

One of the natural consequences of uniprofessional education is that the professional barriers and silos remain and in addition the traditional hierarchical structures are perpetuated.

POLY-Professionals

If we agree that there is a need for a more collaborative approach for all professions in health then a new model is required. The concept of all health care professionals having equal responsibility and accountability for the healthcare system and individuals within it has been argued for (Roff and Dherwani 2011). Roff and Dherwani state that at whatever level we have to function as POLY-professionals we are all responsible for:

Patients and public;

Other health care team members and oneself;

Lifelong learning;

Yourself as a safe, healthy, and honest clinician (Roff and Dherwani 2011).

The concept that as a professional individual one has responsibility for other health care team members is interesting but is not, as yet, supported by regulators. For example in mental health, where Multi-Disciplinary teams (MDTs) in the form of Community Mental Health Teams (CMHTs) were operational in the 1960s GMC guidance (GMC 2013) states that doctors in a mental health team have a responsibility to ensure systems are in place but are not responsible for others' actions. So, POLY as described by Roff and Dhwerwani (2011) is an abstract concept that may not be applicable in the legal framework that health care professionals work.

Multidisciplinary Learning (MDL)

Multidisciplinary learning (MDL) (also known as MD education) involves members of different branches of the same profession. So, within nursing this could be general

nurses, paediatric nurses and advanced nurse practitioners. These two approaches will be referred to these to as MDL.

Multiprofessional Education (MPE)

Multiprofessional education (MPE) or MP learning (MPL) was defined by the World health organisation (WHO 1987) as;

> *the process by which a group of students (or workers) from the health related occupations with different occupational backgrounds learn*

together during certain periods of their education, with interaction as an important goal, to collaborate in improving promotion, preventive, curative, rehabilitative and other health-related services.

Interestingly the WHO's definition of MPL is almost identical to that of IPE published by the Centre for the Advancement of IP Education (CAIPE). A more up to date and accepted definition of MPL (Leathard 1994) distinguishing it from IPE is:

the process by which different professionals come together and achieve the same learning outcomes with the same content.

Then in 2008 the WHO (2010) applied the definition of MDL to their definition of IPE. Therefore, MPL is two or more groups of professionals learning together, side by side mapped to the same learning outcomes. The aim is the successful completion of the same learning outcomes. One example would be psychiatrists and social workers attending the same lecture on the Mental Health Act. Each profession will look at the content from their own perspective without explicit or planned reference to the other profession's roles and responsibilities.

Care Co-ordination

Care co-ordination is another much misused term. In a review (McDonald et al. 2007) 40 different definitions are described. Although these were extremely diverse across many sectors the authors distilled out five key elements that made up care co-ordination:

1 Typically, numerous participants are involved.
2 Participants are dependent on each other to carry out activities that each cannot do alone.
3 In order to carry out the activities there is a need for each party to understand each other's roles and responsibilities and how each interface.
4 All participants rely on sharing knowledge.
5 The aim is to provide appropriate delivery of health care services.
As a result, they have offered a definition (Mc Donald et al. 2007, p. 41):

The deliberate organization of patient care activities between two or more participants (including the patient) involved in a patient's care to facilitate the appropriate delivery of health care services. Organizing care involves the marshalling of personnel and other resources needed to carry out all required patient care activities, and is often managed by the exchange of information among participants responsible for different aspects of care.

Figure 2.1 shows the distinction between profession and discipline. Within the single profession of medicine, there are a number of separate disciplines,

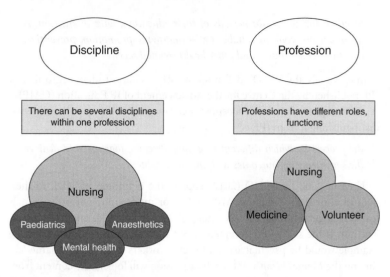

Figure 2.1 Professions and disciplines.

psychiatrist, oncologist and surgeon as examples. Separate professions have boundaries defined by regulators, roles and responsibilities.

The following terms are frequently linked to care co-ordination and for inclusiveness, each will be discussed briefly including:

Teamwork
Continuity of care
Disease management
Case management
Care management
Chronic care model
Care navigator

Teamwork

In the NHS and in other health care systems across the world, Multidisciplinary Teams (MDTs) are seen as a multi professional vehicle for enhancing the delivery of care for patients. MDTs frequently include more than one agency and hence stray into inter-agency and multi-agency working (see later) although, in practice, continue to be referred to as MDTs. Teamwork is required due to the increasing complexity in patient management and subspecialisation of health professionals, particularly in medicine.

Another driver for the development of MDTs has been the changing work patterns across the heath care sector including reduced hours (Wagner 2000).

A systematic review of the cost-effectiveness of MDTs in secondary care (Ke et al. 2013) concluded that there was inconclusive evidence to determine if they were cost-effective or not. A useful working definition of MDTs is provided by NHS England (2014):

> How health and care professionals work together to support people with complex care needs that have been identified through risk stratification and case finding.

Continuity of Care

This is included here as it is frequently used in conjunction with MDTs, care co-ordination and other terms. As with most of these concepts it has many definitions. It could be argued that continuity of care is the individual patient's experience of the level of co-ordination of their care over a period of time, the concept of the right interventions at the right time and in the right order (Haggerty et al. 2003). So it can be seen as the existence of a constant within the patient journey and that could be one single practitioner or group of clinicians that connects different episodes of care.

Disease Management

This is another term that is used to signify a systematic co-ordination of healthcare interventions. It is seen as a process that supports the patient/ clinician relationship with an emphasis on prevention of complication and relapse (Disease Management Association of America 2007).

Case Management

Case management is a general term with no single agreed definition. Care-ordination is usually described as an element within case management (Hutt et al. 2004). The King's Fund describe the core components of a case management programme (Ross et al. 2011) as:

1 *case-finding*
2 *assessment*
3 *care planning*
4 *care co-ordination (usually undertaken by a case manager in the context of a multidisciplinary team). This can include, but is not limited to:*
    i *medication management*
    ii *self-care support*
    iii *advocacy and negotiation*
    iv *psychosocial support*
    v *monitoring and review.*
5 *case closure (in time-limited interventions)*

Although this description appears to describe a sequential pathway, the authors are clear in articulating that this is not the case in the real work of clinical practice.

Care Management (CM)

Care management and care co-ordination are frequently used inter changeably.

Care management has been defined as a set of activities designed to assist patients and their support systems in managing health conditions and related psychosocial problems more effectively, with the aim of improving patients' health status and reducing the need for medical services.

Care management involves providing clinical and support services, including care co-ordination, provided by a nurse or other clinically trained provider. The pattern and type of clinical interventions will vary depending on the nature and complexity of the individual patient's health care needs.

The key components of care management include:

- Identify patients most likely to benefit from care management.
- Assess the risks and needs of each patient.
- Develop a care plan together with the patient/family.
- Teach the patient/family about the diseases and their management, including medication management.
- Coach the patient/family how to respond to worsening symptoms in order to avoid the need for hospital admissions.
- Track how the patient is doing over time.
- Revise the care plan as needed. (Schultz and McDonald 2014)

Care management extends beyond medical issues to address, where possible, how patients' psychosocial circumstances affect their ability to follow treatment recommendations and achieve a healthy lifestyle. The goals are to maintain or improve patients' functional status, increase their capacity to self-manage their condition, eliminate unnecessary clinical testing, and reduce the need for acute care services.

Chronic Care Model

The chronic care model was a term was coined by Wagner (1998) to describe a model for effective care of chronic illness. It has also been described as the guided care model (Boult et al. 2008) who developed a model to meet the growing mismatch between the chronic care needs of the population and the acute care orientation of the health care system.

The chronic care model is a method for ensuring effective care is provided to patients with chronic conditions through a health care delivery system with great emphasis on the systems approach. Therefore, an MDT based in the community would undertake the following:

1 comprehensive assessment.
2 applying an appropriate range of interventions in order to optimise disease control and reduce morbidity; with a focus on well-being.

In this health-care-system links to community services is key.

Care Navigator (Patient Navigator)

There is no widely accepted definition of a care or patient navigator. One definition offered by Dohan and Schrag (2005) is;

> someone who help[s] assist patients overcome barriers to care.

There are a number of examples of the use of patient navigators in the literature, one example in a breast screening service (Battaglia et al. 2007). The aim of using the patient navigator is to improve the outcome for individual patients by helping them to navigate their way through what are extremely complex heath care systems. The navigator helps the patient overcome barriers to accessing care, be that through organising financial support or translation services. This is an example of a patient-centred approach in action.

Interprofessional Collaboration (IPC)

The word 'collaborate' is derived from the Latin 'com' – 'together' – and 'laborare' – 'to work'. There is an inherent duality within this word. It is defined as: to work with others on a joint venture and also, to collaborate with an enemy, for example, to collaborate with an enemy occupying one's country. So, collaboration may be perceived to imply a creative tension and that change on one or both sides will be required for success.

Interprofessional collaboration (IPC) has been defined as:

> The process in which different professional groups work together to positively impact health care. (Zwarenstein et al. 2009)

So, the focus with IPC is working together with an explicit agreement between professionals that values the expertise and contribution that each of the professionals brings to the care of the patient. Challenges that arise in IPC are similar to many interprofessional learning experiences and include: limited understanding of others' roles, power dynamics between professional factions and conflict because of different approaches to the same patient 'problem'.

Within IPC three types of intervention have been described (Goldman et al. 2009):

1 interprofessional education;
2 interprofessional practice;
3 interprofessional organisation interventions.

This review highlights the point that there is a significant overlap between these terms and concepts and it is imperative if one is designing a course or programme that one describes a clear definition of the approach and model underpinning its development. There is much overlap between IPC and shared care (see later). It has also been shown that suboptimal IPC can lead to significant patient safety issues and, in particular, issues in communication between professionals can lead to increased mortality (The Joint Commission 2002).

What can be used to differentiate between a MDT and an IPC scenario? Sheehan et al. (2007) compared the language in a MDT and an IPC team showing that in the latter the language and communication patterns are characterised by inclusive language, continual sharing of information between team members and a collaborative working approach. In the MDT the members worked in parallel and did not have a common understanding of the issues that could influence the outcome for the patient.

Within IPC there are terms such as 'IPC practice-based interventions' defined as strategies operational in health care settings, ward rounds, audit with the aim of improving work interactions and processes between two or more types of professionals. These are essentially the specific interventions used to enhance IPC.

Shared Care

Shared care is another important concept and one definition is:

> The joint participation of primary care physicians and specialty care physicians in the planned delivery of care, informed by an enhanced information exchange over and above routine discharge and referral notices. (Smith et al. 2007)

In this definition the enhanced processes are described as in the interaction between two types of medical physician, in other words, not across different professions.

Interagency Working

Interagency working (IAW) is best seen as a generic term, aligned to multiagency working. There is no generally accepted definition of IAW but one proffered by Lloyd et al. (2001), albeit tentatively is:

> where there is more than one agency working together in a planned and formal way.

Multiagency Working

Multiagency working is a term used to imply a wide range of approaches, structures and processes. Atkinson et al. (2002) describe five different forms of multiagency activity:

1 Decision making groups;
2 Consultation and training;
3 Centre-based delivery;
4 Co-ordinated delivery; and
5 Team operational delivery.

So multiagency working implies more than one agency working with a patient, but not necessarily in a joined up fashion. Most are largely based upon three common principles: information sharing, joint decision-making and co-ordinated intervention. There are models that describe the extent of multiagency working, which lies along a continuum from simple information exchange to full partnership working.

Gaster et al. (1999, p. 9) describe a ladder of partnership the key elements of which are:

• Information exchange;
• Planning action;
• Implementing projects and service plans;
• Co-ordination and co-operation in practice;
• Collaboration and full partnership.

Transprofessional Education

With transprofessional education the MPE takes place in a clinical setting and not in a class room or simulation suite. The learners function as members of a MP team in the delivery of real care to patients.

Interprofessional Learning (Education)

Inteprofessional education (IPE) was defined as:

> *occasions when two or more professions learn with, from and about each other to improve collaboration and quality of care.*
>
> (CAIPE 1997)

Interprofessional learning (IPL) therefore is:

> *Learning arising from interaction between members (or students) of two or more professions. This may be a product of interprofessional education or happen spontaneously in the workplace or in education settings. (Freeth et al. 2005)*

IPL is more than observing a student or clinician from another discipline or profession. The key is all learners engaging in reflection and discussion about similarities and differences between different professions. It is through this process that misconceptions and stereotypes can be addressed and communication skills can be rehearsed. In addition in an ever-changing environment, a complex adaptive system that health and social care reside in, allows each profession to understand better the scope of practice of other professions.

The World Health Organisation offered the following definition of IPE:

> *when students from two or more professions learn about, from and with each other to enable effective collaboration and improve health outcomes.*
> (WHO 2010)

Team-Based Interprofessional Practice Placement

Team-based interprofessional practice placement (TIPP) is a type of clinical placement. The General Medical Council (GMC) as an example of one regulator in the UK has defined this as the placement of a medical student in a working/learning environment that provides health care services to the public (GMC 2011). Brewer and Barr (2016) define TIPP as:

> *A dedicated and prearranged opportunity for a number of students from health, social care and related professions to learn together for a period of time in the same setting as they perform typical activities of their profession as a team focused on a client-centred approach.* (Brewer and Barr 2016, p. 747)

Collaborative Practice

Collaborative practice as defined by the WHO (2010):

> *occurs when multiple health care workers from different professions work together with patients, families to deliver the highest quality of care across settings.* (WHO 2010, p.13)

Human Factors

Human factors is an established scientific discipline used in many other safety-critical sectors such as the aerospace industry.

Human factors in health care has two main aims (i) to support health care professionals and (ii) promote high quality safer care for patients. This approach offers an integrated, evidence-based and co-ordinated methodology to ensure patient safety and facilitate continuous quality improvement.

A definition of human factors within the healthcare setting is offered by Catchpole and McCulloch (2010);

> *Enhancing clinical performance through an understanding of the effects of teamwork, tasks, equipment, workspace, culture and organisation on human behaviour and abilities and application of that knowledge in clinical settings.*

The delivery of health and social care by its very nature takes place in a very pressurised environment. As such, errors will occur and are inevitable. The science of human factors is about designing systems, in this case health care systems that are resilient to unanticipated events, so human factors is not about eliminating human error within this environment.

There is a misconception that human factors training eliminates error by teaching or informing health care staff how to change their behaviour. The reality is that the human factor science addresses the issues of error by modifying the design of the system in which the individuals are operating to aid decision-making and aid the individual people. The key element to human factors work is focusing on factors across the decision-making process, from the individual health care worker level to organisational level. So for example human factors will focus on human physical characteristics, human cognitive characteristics, as well as the human interactions with the entire organisational system, for example how procedural policies, patient workloads can be redesigned to mitigate errors.

Team Training

There are various models of team training and three will be described here as they have been used and reported in Cochrane reviews that are considered amongst other studies in Chapter 3 These are:
1 PRECEDE/PROCEED model;
2 Theory of Planned Behaviour; and
3 The treatment implementation model

PRECEDE/PROCEED Model

This is essentially a comprehensive model for designing and evaluating health systems (Green 1974). The focus is on outcomes as opposed to outputs. With this framework health behaviour is seen as being influenced by individual and environmental factors reflecting the two separate processes in the model. The first is an educational diagnosis (analysis) the PRECEDE being an acronym:

Predisposing,
Reinforcing and
Enabling
Constructs in
Educational
Diagnosis and
Evaluation

The second process is an ecological or 'organisational' diagnosis with the PROCEED being an acronym:

Policy,
Regulatory and
Organisational
Constructs in
Educational and
Environmental
Development

Theory of Planned Behaviour

The theory of planed behaviour (TPB) can be used to identify the variables that determine behaviour (Ajzen 1991). TPB has been widely used in health care settings to explain health care professionals' behaviour (Godin et al. 2008).

TPB postulates that intention to do something is an immediate key determinant of subsequent behaviour. In turn, intention depends on three direct constructs, attitudes, subjective norms and perceived behavioural control. Each of these are influenced by indirect constructs as described in Table 2.1.

Others, (Côté et al. 2012) have added moral norms and past behaviour as additional determinants of behaviour.

So, to change behaviour the introduction of training to influence the indirect constructs will be likely to shift intention in the direction required. For example Côté et al. (2012) concluded that interventions focused on increasing nurses' perceptions that using published evidence is their responsibility will promote or enhance evidence-based nursing and lead to improved care for patients.

The Treatment Implementation Model

This model was the framework of one study (Strasser et al. 2008) discussed in detail in Chapter 3. The model describes three essential components that need to be present to ensure that clinical trials are valid (Lichstein et al. 1994). This model arose out of consideration of the efficacy of psychotherapy interventions but can be used as a framework to ensure any trial, for example an educational intervention, is valid.

Table 2.1 Direct and indirect constructs.

Direct construct	Indirect construct
Attitude	Behavioural beliefs
Subjective norms	Normative beliefs
Perceived behavioural controls	Control beliefs

The three components are delivery, receipt and enactment. Lichstein et al. (1994) argue that each of these three needs to be fully implemented and that the researchers' role is to ensure that all three are completed equally. In order to achieve this there needs to be a full assessment of each of these elements built into the protocol.

Plan Do Study Act (PDSA)

The Plan Do Study Act (PDSA) model (Deming 1986) was used in one referenced study Barceló et al. 2010 (see Chapter 3). For completeness, a brief description will be offered.

The PDSA cycle is a frequently used tool for continuous quality improvement. The first step is to…

Plan … what is the problem that needs addressed?

> How does one know it is a problem?
>
> What is the overall aim?
>
> What are the specific objectives?
>
> Baseline measurements are needed … the, where are we now?

Do … carry out the intervention

> Take measurements over a period of time

Study … study or analyse the data.

> Was the outcome close to that projected?
>
> Where there any unintended consequences?
>
> Where there any lessons to be learnt?

Act … ensure that any improvements are enacted on

The evidence suggests that the PDSA cycle approach works best with small incremental changes to systems with repeating cycles.

Chapter Summary

This chapter offers a brief summary of definitions of key terms to help the reader get to grips with the wide range of terms that are often used interchangeably in the IPE literature. This interchangeability can lead to confusion.

The historical perspective of the term profession is explored together with broader concepts such as care in the community, partnership working, team working and human factors.

Specific processes that have been used in some of the published evaluation studies that will be explored in depth in Chapter 3 are also defined such as the PDSA cycle and the PRECEDE/PROCEED model.

The key concept in IPE is to learn with, from and about each other to enhance collaborative practice to improve the quality of care to patients. One risk in badly designed IPE learning experiences is that the different professions participating focus solely on acquiring the same knowledge or skills. The real difference with IPE is that they learn from each other and learn *about* each others' roles, skills and attitudes.

So, in IPE learners from various professions learn together as a team. Their collaborative interaction is characterised by the integration and modification of different professions' contributions in light of the input from other professions.

The unique feature of IPE is the type of cognitive and behavioural change that occurs: participants understand the core principles and concepts of each contributing discipline and are familiar with the basic language and mind sets of the various disciplines. Prior to participating in IPE students must have basic knowledge and skills related to their own profession.

IPE programmes can have many different types of aims and each learning experience has to be tailored with the learning outcomes in mind, as with any learning.

References

Ajzen, I. (1991). The theory of planned behaviour. *Organizational Behaviour and Human Decision Processes* 50: 79–211.

Atkinson, M., Wilkin, A., Stott, A. et al. (2002). *Multi-Agency Working: A Detailed Study*. Slough: National Foundation for Education Research.

Audit Commission (1986). *Making a Reality of Community Care*. HMSO.

Audit Commission (1998). *A Fruitful Partnership: Effective Partnership Working*. London: HMSO.

Barceló, A., Cafiero, E., de Boer, M. et al. (2010). Using collaborative learning to improve diabetes care and outcomes: the VIDA project. *Primary Care Diabetes* 4 (3): 145–153.

Barr, H. (2002). *Interprofessional Education Today, Yesterday and Tomorrow; A Review*. London: Learning and Teaching support Network, Centre for Health Sciences and Practice.

Barr, H., Koppel, I., Reeves, S. et al. (2005). *Effective Interprofessional Education: Argument, Assumption and Evidence*. Oxford: Blackwell Publishing.

Battaglia, T.A., Roloff, K., Posner, M.A. et al. (2007). Improving follow up to abnormal breast cancer screening in an urban population: a patient navigation intervention. *Cancer* 109 (2 Suppl): 359–367.

Boult, C., Karm, I., and Groves, C. (2008). Improving chronic care: the 'guided Care' model. *The Permanente Journal* 12 (1): 50–54.

Brewer, M.L. and Barr, H. (2016). Interprofessional education and practice guide no. 8: team-based interprofessional practice placement. *Journal of Interprofessional Care* 30 (6): 747–753.

CAIPE (1997). Interprofessional Education – A Definition. CAIPE Bulletin No. 13.

Campbell, J. and Johnson, C. (1999). Trend spotting; fashions in medical education. *British Medical Journal* 322: 676.

Carlton, N., Ritchie, J. and Harriss, K. (2003). Cross-Boundary issues in Homelessness Services for People with Multiple Needs. Unpublished research report for Bristol City Council, Bath and North East Somerset Council, South Gloucestershire Council and North Somerset Council. Bristol: University of the West of England.

Catchpole, K. and McCulloch, P. (2010). Human factors in critical care: towards standardized integrated human-centred systems of work. *Current Opinion in Critical Care* 16 (6): 618–622. https://doi.org/10.1097/MCC.0b013e32833e9b4b.

Côté, F., Gagnon, J., Houme, P.K. et al. (2012). Using the theory of planned behaviour to predict nurses' intention to integrate research evidence into clinical decision-making. *Journal of Advanced Nursing* 68 (10): 2289–2298.

Cohen, J.J. (2007). Linking professionalism to humanism; what it means, why it matters. *Academic Medicine* 82: 1029–1032.

Cruess, R., Cruess, S., and Johnson, S.E. (1999). Renewing professionalism: an opportunity for medicine. *Academic Medicine* 74 (8): 878–884.

Cruess, R.L. and Cruess, S.R. (2008). Expectations and obligations: professionalism and medicine's social contract with society. *Perspectives in Biology and Medicine* 51: 579–588.

Disease Management Association of America (2007). Definition of Disease Management. https://diseasemanagementassociationofamericawpan.wordpress.com/ (accessed: 30 June 2018).

Dohan, D. and Schrag, D. (2005). Using navigators to improve care of underserved patients: current practices and approaches. *Cancer* 104 (4): 848–855.

Emanuel, L.I. (2004). Deriving professionalism from its roots. *American Journal of Bioethics* 4 (2): 17–18.

Francis, R. (2013). *Mid Staffordshire NHS Foundation Trust Public Inquiry*. London: Stationery Office.

Freeth, D., Hammick, M., Reeves, S. et al. (2005). *Effective Interprofessional Education: Development, Delivery and Evaluation*. Oxford: Blackwell.

Gaster, L., Deakin, N. and Riseborough, M. (1999). History, Strategy or Lottery? The realities of Local Government /Voluntary Sector Relations. London: Improvement and Development Agency (IdeA).

General Medical Council (2011). Clinical placements for medical students. https://www.gmc-uk.org/-/media/documents/clinical-placements-for-medical-students---guidance-0815_pdf-56437824.pdf (accessed: 30 June 2018).

General Medical Council (2013). Accountability in multi-disciplinary and multi-agency mental health teams. https://www.gmc-uk.org/-/media/ethical-guidance/related-pdf-items/leadership-and-management/accountability-in-multi-disciplinary-teams.pdf (accessed: 30 June 2018).

General Pharmaceutical Council (2017). Standards for pharmacy professionals. https://www.pharmacyregulation.org/sites/default/files/standards_for_pharmacy_professionals_may_2017_0.pdf (accessed: 30 June 2018).

Goldman, J., Zwarenstein, M., Bhattacharyya, O. et al. (2009). Improving the clarity of the interprofessional field: implications for research and continuing interprofessional education. *Journal of Continuing Education in the Health Professions* 29 (3): 151–156.

Godin, G., Belanger-Gravel, A., Eccles, M. et al. (2008). Healthcare professionals' intentions and behaviours: a systematic review of studies based on social cognitive theories. *Implementation Science* 3: 36.

Green, L.W. (1974). Towards cost-benefit evaluations of health education: some concepts, methods, and examples. *Health Education Monographs* 2 (Suppl. 2): 34–64.

Haggerty, J.L., Reid, R.J., Freeman, G.K. et al. (2003). Continuity of care: a multidisciplinary review. *British Medical Journal* 327 (7425): 1219–1221.

Hilton, S. and Slotnick, H.B. (2005). Proto-professionalism: how professionalism occurs across the continuum of medical education. *Medical Education* 39 (1): 58–65.

Hutt, R., Rosen, R., and McCauley, J. (2004). *Case-Managing Long-Term Conditions: What Impact Does it Have in the Treatment of Older People?* London: The Kings Fund.

Ke, M.K., Blazeby, J.M., Strong, S. et al. (2013). Are multidisciplinary teams in secondary care cost-effective? A systematic review of the literature. *Cost Effectiveness and Resource Allocation* 11: 7.

Laming, L. (2003). *Inquiry into the Death of Victoria Climbié*. London: The Stationery Office.

Leathard, A. (ed.) (1994). Interprofessional developments in Britain: an overview. In: *Going Inter-Professional: Working Together for Health and Welfare*, 3–37. London: Routledge.

Lichstein, K.L., Riedel, B.W., and Grieve, R. (1994). Fair tests of clinical trials: a treatment implementation model. *Advances in Behaviour Research Therapy* 16: 1–29.

Lloyd, G., Stead, J., and Kendrick, A. (2001). *Hanging on in There; A Study of Interagency Working to Prevent School Exclusion*. London: National Childrens' Bureau/Joseph Rowntree Foundation.

NHS England (2014). MDT Development – Working toward an effective multidisciplinary/multiagency team. http://www.england.nhs.uk/wp-content uploads/2015/01/mdt-dev-guid-flat-fin.pdf (accessed: 17 June 2018).

Nursing and Midwifery Council (2015).*The Code*. Professional standards of practice and behaviour for nurses and midwives. www.nmc.org.uk/standards/code (accessed: 30 June 2018).

Powell, M. and Glendinning, C. (2002). Introduction. In: *Partnerships, New Labour and the Governance of Welfare* (ed. C. Glendinning, M. Powell and K. Rummery), 1–14. Bristol: The Policy Press.

Roff, S. and Dherwani, K. (2011). Development of inventory for polyprofessionalism lapses at the proto-professional stage of health professions education together with recommended responses. *Medical Teacher* 33 (3): 239–243.

Rosen, R. and Dewar, S. (2004). *On Being a Doctor; Redefining Medical Professionalism for Better Patient Care*. London: The Kings's Fund.

Ross, S., Curry, N., and Goodwin, N. (2011). *Case Management. What It is and How it Can Best be Implemented*. London: The Kings Fund.

Schultz, E.M. and McDonald, K.M. (2014). What is care coordination? *International Journal of Care Coordination* 17: 5–24.

Sheehan, D., Robertson, L., and Ormond, T. (2007). Comparison of language used and patterns of communication in interprofessional and multidisciplinary teams. *Journal of Interprofessional Care* 21 (1): 17–30.

Smith, J. (2004). *The Shipman Inquiry*. London: Stationery Office.

Smith, S.M., Allwright, S., and O'Dowd, T. (2007). Effectiveness of shared care across the interface between primary and speciality care in chronic disease management. *Cochrane Database of Systematic Reviews* 2007 (3): 1–56.

Sox, C.H. (2007). The ethical foundations of professionalism; a sociological history. *Chest* 131: 1532–1540.

Strasser, D.C., Falconer, J.A., Stevens, A.B. et al. (2008). Team training and stroke rehabilitation outcomes: a cluster randomized trial. *Archives of Physical Medicine Rehabilitation* 89: 10–15.

The Joint Commission (2002). Sentinel Event Alert: Delays in treatment. The Joint Commission 2002, issue 26 June 17.

Wagner, E.,.H. (2000). The role of patient care teams in chronic disease management. *British Medical Journal* 320 (7234): 569–572.

World Health Organisation (1987). Learning together to work together for health, Report of a WHO Study group on the Multiprofessional Education of Health Personnel: the Team Approach, Technical Report Series 769, Geneva: World Health Organisation.

World Health Organization (2010). *Framework for Action on Interprofessional & Collaborative Practice*. Geneva: World Health Organisation.

Zwarenstein, M., Goldman, J., and Reeves, S. (2009). Interprofessional collaboration: effects of practice-based interventions on professional practice and healthcare outcomes. *Cochrane Database of Systematic Reviews* (3): 1–29.

McDonald, K.M., Sundaram, V., Bravata, D.M. et al. (2007). *Care Coordination*, Closing the Quality Gap: A Critical Analysis of Quality Improvement Strategies. Technical Review 9.7. Rockville, MD: Agency for Healthcare Research and Quality.

Wagner, E.H. (1998). Chronic disease management: what will it take to improve care for chronic illness? *Effective Clinical Practice* 1 (1): 2–4.

Deming, W.E. (1986). *Out of the crisis*. Center for Advanced Engineering Study: MIT Press.

Chapter 3 Interprofessional Education – Evidence It Works

In today's environment with the need to demonstrate value for money, irrespective of the sector, but particularly in the hard pressed health arena, a key question is … Does Interprofessional Education (IPE) work? Is it still the case that nurses prefer learning with their peers and doctors with doctors? Therefore, there needs to be a certain level of evidence that IPE works, and works for patients, not just for the staff.

This chapter will review some of the published work in this field. The level of evidence for the effectiveness of IPE interventions varies from randomised controlled trials to descriptive and exploratory studies. The levels of evaluation also have a wide range and include improvement to patient care, perception and understanding of other professionals.

Harden's Ladder

In considering any studies that attempt to investigate the effectiveness of IPE it is useful to use re-visit Harden's ladder (Harden 2000) in order to map or at least to attempt to map across. As will become apparent, the educational interventions reported in a wide range of studies utilise a diverse array of teaching methods, not all of which easily sit with the IPE arena.

To recap, the particular approaches that can be used lie along a continuum with Isolation at one end to Trans-disciplinary at the other. Harden described these as 11 steps in multiprofessional education. These can be used to benchmark any teaching/learning experience.

Harden's 11 steps:

1 Isolation
2 Awareness
3 Harmonisation

How to Succeed at Interprofessional Education, First Edition. Peter Donnelly.
© 2019 John Wiley & Sons Ltd. Published 2019 by John Wiley & Sons Ltd.

4 Nesting
5 Temporal co-ordination
6 Sharing
7 Correlation
8 Complementary
9 Multi-disciplinary
10 Inter-disciplinary
11 Trans-disciplinary

Harden devised the ladder as a means to facilitate integration in curricula. He describes that as one moves up the ladder there is less focus on the separate disciplines or professions but an increasing need for integration. The previous SPICES model (Harden et al. 1984) for curricula integration is represented as a continuum with single discipline teaching at one end and full integration at the other. Harden's view was that as one moves up the ladder that there was a greater need for staff participation in the design and delivery of the curriculum, hence the ladder could be useful for any organisation to help in planning. Each of these levels is a description essentially based on the level of collaboration. It must be remembered, that each is an appropriate teaching strategy depending on the specific aims and objectives of the course or programme.

Isolation

This is the scenario where each profession organises it's own learning and is completely unaware of what is learnt by any other professions and does not take any steps to learn of others. This is the extreme end of the uniprofessional education (UPE) spectrum. An example would be a short two-hour course with the learning objective of each first year trainee in surgery being able to suture a scalp laceration. That is a specific procedural task that does not and is not likely to require any other clinician to be involved. Hence, an UPE approach could be argued to be appropriate.

Awareness

At this level, each profession has a level of awareness of each other's roles and this may be referred to in the teaching or training but there is no formal collaboration between the different professions.

Harmonisation

At this level there is some discussion and consultation between the professions in regard to the design of the learning. This may be reflected in more explicit reference to each other's roles. In this scenario the programme remains UPE but with a greater level of acknowledgement of other professionals roles and contributions.

Nesting

At this level, we are moving closer to more involvement in a planned fashion of other professions in the design and delivery of the learning. However, the main focus is still UPE with the second (other) professions contributing to just one aspect on the learning, for example within a medical school module on clinical skills in psychiatry a community pharmacist provides a two day placement for students.

Temporal Co-ordination

With this level, the two or more professional groups share in the learning programme but there is no planned collaboration between them. An element of joint planning of the learning is required but this is at a superficial level only. Any collaboration is by chance and not by design. An example is learners from two or more professions attending the same lecture. In this scenario the unplanned IPE may occur as a result of the informal networking, but is not planned. This form of unplanned IPE is extremely valuable as an unintended consequence.

Sharing

Moving along the continuum, we have the next step, shared teaching. This is where there is planned interaction between the different professionals as a part of the programme. This shared learning/collaboration at this level, refers to only one well-demarcated aspect of the programme. So the programme as a whole is UPE with one aspect where collaboration exists.

Correlation

This stage refers to a further step into a more planned multi-professional (MP) perspective with regular, well defined MP sessions embedded in a UP programme.

Complimentary

This stage is where there is almost equal emphasis on UP and MP with each aspect or approach complementing the other.

Multi-disciplinary

At this level, the emphasis on UPE all but disappears with the focus on a multi-disciplinary approach. However each profession discusses the 'problem', in the scenario of Problem Based Learning, from it's own perspective. So the learners learn by addressing a jointly owned problem together, but from the perspective of their own profession.

Inter-disciplinary

With this stage, all learners look at the problem with the other profession's perspective as well as their own. So in a role play scenario, for example, the nurse may 'play' the physiotherapist. Learning is focused on the objective of enhancing collaborative practice. So, there is common content but with the similarities and differences in approach between the professions explored and discussed in a planned fashion.

Trans-disciplinary

In this stage, the MPE takes place in the context of clinical practice. The environment is not a classroom but in real practice settings. An example is the University of Limburg (Wahlstrom and Sanden 1998) where all professions learn together in clinical IPE wards as active working participants.

Using Harden's ladder can be a useful reference point when considering or analysing any learning. It can also be used as one element to gather a clear picture of where your programme lies or where it could lie. As such, this can then be used as a baseline for design and for considering what steps you might want to take to move the learning from say nesting, to the next level or decide that for your learners nesting is an appropriate strategy at this point.

Although useful to some extent, Harden's ladder has limited usefulness in practice as an assessment tool.

Barr (1996) described a number of different dimensions of IPE that can also be used. These are explored in detail in Chapter 6.

A framework described by Xyrichis et al. (2017) offers a more or potentially more useful approach. Please see Chapter 5 for more detail.

The Evidence for Effectiveness of IPE Interventions

In this section two Cochrane reviews will be examined in some detail; (i) Reeves et al. (2013) and (ii) Reeves et al. (2017).

It is important to understand the methodology and in particular the aims and subsequent search strategy used by Reeves et al. (2013) in their Cochrane review of the effectiveness of IPE.

There were two stated objectives:

… to assess the effectiveness of IPE compared to;

1 separate, profession specific education interventions; and
2 control groups which received no education intervention.

The types of study included were randomised controlled trials (RCTs), controlled before and after (CBA) and time interrupted studies (TISs).

The eligibility criteria for participants was broadly defined as all health and social care professionals. The types of interventions included all types of education, training and learning which involved more than one profession in joint interactive learning. The authors defined an IPE intervention as follows:

> *An IPE intervention occurs when members of more than one health or social care (or both) profession learn interactively together, for the explicit purpose of improving interprofessional collaboration or the health/ well being (or both) of patients/clients. Interactive learning requires active learner participation, and active exchange between learners from different professions.* (Reeves et al. 2013, p. 5)

Randomised Controlled Trials

The randomised controlled trial (RCT) is one of the simplest, but most scientific, methodologies to test hypotheses (Stolberg et al. 2004). In essence, the RCT is a study in which subjects are allocated at random to receive one of several interventions. In the IPE context, the term 'intervention' refers to educational interventions.

The randomisation process gives the RCT its strength resulting in all subjects having the same chance of being assigned to each of the study groups. The purpose of random allocation of subjects is to ensure that the characteristics of the participants are as likely to be as similar as possible across groups at the start of the comparison (also called the baseline). This reduces the risk of a serious imbalance in known and unknown factors that could influence the outcome.

Reeves et al. (2013) identified eight studies that meet the criteria for this study type. These studies will be described and critiqued in this section.

Barceló et al. (2010) reported on a RCT involving 43 primary care teams based in 10 public health centres in Veracruz state, in Mexico. The subjects included teams made up of physicians, nurses and some of the teams included nutritionists and psychologists. The number and detailed professional profiles in each team were not described.

Ten health teams were randomly allocated to receive either the intervention or no intervention. The intervention itself consisted of the teams participating in three learning sessions over a period of 18 months. The educational strategy is described as having three elements;
1 a structured patient diabetes education programme
2 training in foot care
3 in-service training for primary care personnel in diabetes management
The educational methodology used included the teams selecting specific objectives to be the subject of Plan Do Study Act (PDSA) improvement cycles

(see Chapter 2 for more detail on PDSA). The learning objectives were identified via problems highlighted within the practice of each of the health centres.

Outcome measures included clinical observations of metabolic control, for example, cholesterol levels and adherence to clinical protocols including periodic foot and eye examinations.

The results indicated that there was a significant difference in glycaemic control in those patients of the intervention group (28% compared to 39%) after intervention (p value 0.05). In addition the proportion of patients achieving 3 or more quality improvement goals increased from 16.6% to 69.7% (p < 0.001) in the intervention group compared to the control group which showed a non-significant decrease from 12.4% to 5.9% (p = 0.118). The number of patients in the intervention group was 196 and in the usual care group was 111.

In this study, although the outcomes for patients were good but the extent of IPE strategies and professional profiles were not detailed.

Brown et al. (1999) reported an RCT with the aim of determining whether a communication skills programme increased patient satisfaction with ambulatory, medical care visits. The study involved 69 primary care physicians, surgeons, medical subspecialties, physician assistants and nurse practitioners from the Permanente Medical Group in Oregon, USA.

Of the circa 1000 eligible subjects 69 volunteered to participate and were randomly assigned to either the intervention group (n = 37) or the control group (n = 32). The intervention consisted of two four-hour workshops one month apart with each participant required to audiotape a minimum of two consultations with patients in between the two workshops.

The workshops comprised brief didactic elements with role-playing to practice communication skills. The evaluation used the Art of Medicine survey measuring patients' self-reported rating of the clinicians' communication skills. The areas covered in the survey are:

How COURTEOUS was the doctor?
How well did the doctor UNDERSTAND your problem?
How well did the doctor EXPLAIN to you what he or she was doing and why?
Did the doctor USE WORDS that were easy for you to understand?
How well did the doctor LISTEN to your concerns and questions?
Did the doctor SPEND ENOUGH time with you?
How much CONFIDENCE do you have in the doctor's ability or competence?
OVERALL, how satisfied are you with the service that you received from the doctor? (Art of medicine survey, www.healthcareresearch.com)

The authors report that this intervention did not improve patient satisfaction scores and concluded that to have an impact on patient satisfaction, more intensive educational interventions are need with a focus on a broader range of skills.

This study involved small numbers and the brief intervention used is not adequately described in terms of the focus or model of IPE utilised. In addition, the ratio of doctors to non-doctors (32/7) does call into question the balance of representation of the different professionals in the teaching sessions.

Campbell et al. (2001) undertook an RCT evaluating a team training approach for emergency departments (EDs) in Pennsylvania and California, USA. The aim was to assess the effectiveness of a system change training programme in improving EDs' staff knowledge of and attitude to domestic violence as well as patient satisfaction and improved identification rates.

Of 39 hospitals within a 100 mile radius of either Pittsburgh or San Francisco 12 were randomly selected and allocated to either intervention group (n = 6 EDs) and control group (n = 6 EDs). Each intervention ED was asked to send a team comprising a doctor, nurse, social worker, and administrator to the training programme. In addition an anonymous staff survey was administered pre and post study, at baseline (n = 3360) and post intervention (n = 313). The survey measured staff attitudes to domestic violence and knowledge. Follow up data were collected at 9–12 months and 18–24 months.

The intervention group received a two-day team training programme. The first day comprised a combination of didactic teaching, role playing of assessment and intervention scenarios with the second day dedicated to system change with the team devising a written action plan/protocol.

Of the six intervention EDs only one sent the full team of physician, nurse, social worker, and administer. Two EDs did not send a physician and five sent a social worker.

The intervention hospitals showed significantly higher levels on systems change indicators (protocols, checklists for example) and higher levels of patient satisfaction than the control groups.

There was no significant difference in the identification rates for battered women using a review of medical records. The authors acknowledged that although protocols and information for women had improved in the experimental groups that actual practice change is more difficult to achieve.

The professional profile of the intervention teams varied significantly and the details of the IPE teaching methods were not described except to state that team training was the approach used.

Nielsen et al. (2007) described a cluster RCT evaluating the effect of team training on the occurrence of adverse outcomes and the process of care in hospital-based labour wards.

Seven hospitals were randomised to the intervention group teamwork training curriculum with eight hospitals acting as controls.

All women pregnant (20–43 weeks gestation) admitted to the hospitals over a 45 month period were included in the study (n = 28 536 deliveries). Baseline data was collected two months pre study and at four months post intervention.

The intervention was based on a teamwork training curriculum (MedTeams Labor & Delivery Team Coordination Course; Locke et al. 2001), with principles based on crew management. The learning consisted of three days of instructor training with four hours of didactic lessons, video scenarios and interactive team training, team structure, problem solving, communication, team skills, workload management and conflict resolution skills. A total of 1307 staff were trained but no detail of discipline or professional background or demographics is reported.

Measurements included maternal and foetal/neonatal outcomes using an Adverse Outcome Index defined as the number of patients with one or more adverse outcomes divided by the total number of deliveries. Process measures included time from registration on the ward to initiation of assessment, time from decision to undertake immediate Caesarean Section (CS) to time of incision and similar time/process measures.

There was no significant difference in the mean Adverse Outcome Index between the intervention and control groups at baseline or post intervention. The only process measure to differ significantly was time from decision to perform an immediate CS, 33 minutes for the control vs 21 minutes for the intervention group (p = 0.3).

The authors conclude that the intervention did not translate to measurable impacts on adverse outcomes. Although the sample sizes were significant, the details of the training programme did not indicate the exact teaching techniques that were used in the team training.

Helitzer et al. (2011) reported on a RCT of communication training of primary care providers with the aim of improving patient centeredness and health risk communication. The participants included physicians, physician assistants and nurse practitioners. Twenty-six eligible providers participated in the study and were randomised to receive the intervention or to act as a control. To further control for the previous finding that female physicians and primary care physicians have superior communication skills the randomisation process was stratified by gender and specialty.

The intervention group comprised six Family Physicians (FP), four Internal Medicine Physicians (IMPs), and two Physician Assistants (PAs) or Nurse Practitioners (NPs). The control group comprised eight FPs, four IMPs, and two PAs/NPs.

The educational intervention consisted of training with three components.
1 A full day training.
2 Individualised feedback on videotaped interactions using simulated patients.
3 Workshops to reinforce strategies for patient engagement.

All providers participated in two or more sets of interactions with real patients where patient-physician communication was independently assessed. Data was collected at 6 and 18 months post intervention.

The results indicated that the intervention group at 6 and 18 months showed a significant difference in scores for patient centeredness ($p < 0.01$ at 6 months and $p = 0.032$ at 18 months).

The description of the educational intervention does not provide detail of the IPE strategies used so it is difficult to gauge the level of IPE used. Although a detailed breakdown in terms of professionals' representation is given there are two issues with this study; (i) there were small numbers in total in the control and intervention groups and (ii) in both the majority were doctors, albeit with a range of disciplines from within medicine. The doctors/PA to nurse ratios were 12/2 in the control and 10/2 in intervention groups again raising the question of the balance of the learning groups professionally.

Strasser et al. (2008) reported on a cluster randomised trial testing whether a team training intervention in the field of stroke rehabilitation is associated with improved patient outcomes.

The subjects included 237 clinical staff in 16 control teams and 227 in 15 intervention teams. The control teams only received online information on effective team functioning while the intervention teams had the same online information and the intervention. The total number of stroke patients treated by these teams before and after intervention was 487.

The intervention teams were stated as comprising the following professional groups: medicine, nursing, occupational therapy, speech language pathology, physical therapists and case managers/social workers. No detail is provided regarding the numerical balance of these professions in either the control or intervention groups.

The intervention was in three phases. In the first, the teams participated in a two-and-a-half day team training workshop targeting two self-identified team leaders from each of the 15 intervention sites. The design and delivery of the team training was guided by the treatment implementation process described by Lichstein et al. (1994) (see Chapter 2 for more detail on this approach).

It is reported that physicians or osteopaths were the most commonly represented discipline amongst team leaders but others included nurses, occupational therapists, social workers, speech language pathologists and administrators.

The second phase of the intervention occurred three to five weeks after the initial workshop, and consisted of action plans to address team process problems based on discussions within the phase 1 workshop. In the third phase (at months three to six) workshop participants received telephone and video conference consultations giving advice on how to implement plans.

Patient outcome data included functional improvement, community discharge and length of stay (LOS). Data was gathered from 487 patients treated by these teams before and after interventions. The results indicated a significant improvement in functional outcome between the intervention and control groups ($p = 0.3038$). There was no significant difference for the other two outcome measures.

The authors concluded that stroke patients treated by a different range of professionals who had participated in a team training programme were significantly more likely to make functional gains than those treated by staff receiving just the online information.

From an IPE research design perspective, there were a wide range of professionals in both control and intervention groups but no detailed breakdown to clarify an equal balance.

Thompson et al. (2000a) described a group RCT in a sample of 60 primary care practices in a health district in England. The aim was to test whether there was a change in the recognition of and recovery from depression. Of the potential 232 practices in the county of Hampshire, 59 practices (169 physicians) were randomly assigned.

The intervention group received an education package provided in two parts. The first part included each practice receiving four hours of seminar (small group work of up to 20 participants in each) supplemented by video tapes to demonstrate interviewing and counselling skills, small group discussion and role play as appropriate. For the second element, the educators remained available to the practice for nine months after the seminars. The control group through this study period did not receive any additional educational intervention.

The subjects within the intervention practices included physicians ($n = 58$) and practice nurses ($n = 64$). Practices in the control group received the education intervention after the study had been completed.

Data was collected at six weeks and six months after patient visits. The results indicated no significant differences between the intervention and control groups in regard to recognition of depression and/or improvement using the Hospital Anxiety and Depression Scale (Zigmond and Snaith 1983). The authors concluded that although this intervention was well received the intervention did not show improvement in either recognition or recovery from depression.

In this study, participants were approximately equally doctors and practice nurses. The nature of the education intervention included small group work supported by video tapes demonstrating communication skills so it is difficult to clarify the level of IPE used. Also, the use of lager small groups of up to 20 participants is questionable when one considers the published work suggesting the optimal size of small groups is of the order of fewer than 10.

Thompson et al. (2000b) reported on a group-randomised study of five primary care clinics from the Group Health Co-operative of Puget Sound, USA. The aim was to test the effect of an intensive intervention to improve asking about domestic violence (DV), case finding and management in primary care.

The intervention was two separate half day training sessions based on the PRECEDE/PROCEED model for behaviour change (see Chapter 2 for more detail). The focus was on changing practitioners predisposing factors (knowledge and attitude for example), enabling factors (system process) and reinforcing factors such as the use of feedback. It is stated that the training was focused on skill building and empowering teams to verbally ask about DV. The intervention was described in more detail in a previous publication (Thompson et al. 1998) and consisted of two training sessions.

The first session provided basic information and used stop-start teaching videos exploring how DV may play out in a clinical setting. In addition participants engaged in team role play (playing their own professional roles) with the aim of clarifying each other's role. The focus of the second session was using role play to build skills in assessing and managing DV.

Two of the five clinics were randomly assigned to the intervention and the other three acted as controls. The intervention group had total 91 participants with the following professional breakdown:

Doctors 29 (31.9%)

Physician assistants 7 (7.7%)

Registered nurses 26 (28.6%)

Licenced practice nurse/medical assistants 29 (31.9%)

Baseline measures were taken before, at 9 months and at 21 months post intervention. A survey was used to assess the outcome measures of knowledge, attitudes and beliefs about DV, self-efficacy, fear of causing offence if asking questions and received after asking questions.

Results at 9 and 21 months showed increased self-efficacy, reduced fear of asking and increased self-perception of asking (not this at 21 months).

Documented asking about DV increased by 14.3% (3.9 fold) and case finding increased by 1.3 fold.

The authors concluded that the intervention improved documented asking about DV, and showed a small increase in case finding.

The participant profile shows a range of professionals but the educational intervention using the PRECEDE/PROCEED model is more closely aligned to change management processes. However, the educational interventions were focused on using role play and interaction between members to rehearse and build skill. On a positive note, there is a clear objective of each team member understanding their own and others' role in order to improve outcomes for patients.

Controlled Before and After Studies (CBA)

The simplest way to evaluate an intervention is to compare outcomes before and after implementation of the intervention. This method is known as an uncontrolled before-after study. The term uncontrolled is used to distinguish this design from a controlled before-after (CBA) study in which the before-after effect of implementation in the intervention group is compared to a control group that has no intervention. With the recent emphasis on improvements in health care delivery in particular, the number of uncontrolled before-after studies is increasing. In CBA studies outcomes are measured before and after a treatment in a group that receives the treatment, and in another group that does not receive the treatment, or that receives a different treatment. However, CBA studies typically have a high risk of bias because of other differences between the groups that are being compared (confounders).

Janson et al. (2009) reported a non-randomised parallel group clinical trial of 384 adult patients with type 2 diabetes. These patients were receiving care in two different General Internal Medicine clinics within the University of California. The patient intervention group (n = 221) received care based on the Improving Chronic Illness Care model (ICIC) model from teams of interprofessional clinical leaders. The control group (n = 163) received traditional care from internal medicine residents. All patients were followed up prospectively for a period an 18 months from 2002 to 2003. The aim was to assess the impact of the interprofessional team care compared with the traditional care on:

1 processes of care;
2 clinical status; and
3 health care utilisation.

The intervention team members participated in the chronic illness curriculum which took place half a day a week for varying periods dependent on the placement length of the different professions. The participants in the intervention teams comprised; four to five medical residents; two nurse practitioner students and two pharmacy students. The control group of patients received the usual care from internal medicine residents.

The education intervention comprised a 60 minute didactic presentation, a 30 minute clinical discussion and 2.5 hours of clinic visits with patients.

The ICIC model is described as having six key elements:

Community resources and policies

Heath care organisations

Self-management support

Delivery system design

Decision support

Clinical information systems

The authors reported that the intervention patients more frequently received assessments such as blood pressure and more planned general medicine visits than the control group. Their conclusions were that the interprofessional team care was effective in improving the quality of care for patients with diabetes treated in General Medical clinics (in addition the other assessments included glycosylated haemoglobin ($p = 0.01$) blood pressure ($p = 0.08$) microalbuminuria ($p = 0.05$) smoking status assessment ($p = 0.02$) and foot exams ($p = 0.0005$).

This study comprised small teams of three health professionals working in a team, doctors, nurses and pharmacy trainees/students. The educational intervention was based on the ICIC model that has elements of teamwork.

Morey et al. (2002) reported a prospective multi-centre evaluation using a quasi-experimental untreated control group design. The aim was to evaluate collaborative behaviour of hospital ED staff.

Nine hospital EDs self-selected to receive either the educational intervention (6 EDs with 684 clinicians) or to act as a control group (3 EDs with 374 clinicians). The intervention was based on an Emergency Team Co-ordination Course (ETCC) organised around five team dimensions, which formed the modules in the curriculum (Risser et al. 1999);

1 Maintain team structure and climate

2 Apply problem solving strategies

3 Communicate with the team

4 Execute plans and manage workload

5 Improve team skills

The intervention comprised eight hours of instruction delivered to these dimensions. Each module consisted of clinical lectures and discussion of each of the team behaviours supported by vignettes taken from real examples. The control group departments received the intervention post assessment.

The participants were physicians, nurses and technicians. The teaching methods used small groups of mixed professionals of up to 16 members. The exact balance of each professional in each of the learning groups was not described.

Data was collected at two four-monthly intervals following the training. The authors reported that the staff who participated in the IPE team-working training programme showed a statistically significant improvement in the quality of observed team behaviours compared to the control group (p = 0.012). In addition the clinical error rate was significantly decreased in the intervention group from 30.9% to 4.4% (p = 0.039).

The authors concluded that their results showed the effectiveness of formal team work training for improving team behaviours, reducing clinical errors and improving staff attitude amongst staff in the ED departments.

With this study a high level curriculum is described and teaching methods included small group work. The exact level of IPE utilised is difficult to gauge. Although the three groups of professional are described an exact break down in terms of profile is not described.

Rask et al. (2007) reported on a quality improvement project to evaluate the effectiveness of a falls management programme in nursing homes. The setting of the study was nursing homes in Georgia, USA.

The study group consisted of 19 nursing home teams with 23 homes as controls. Each study home was asked to select an interdisciplinary falls team to include: a physical or occupational therapist; two to four certified nursing assistants; maintenance staff and a Director of nursing.

These teams participated in a falls management programme (FMP) consisting of a one day interactive workshop followed by a second workshop one month later in order to address any challenges that had arisen. The focus in the workshops was on the team's development of problem-solving skills to enhance the weekly monitoring and selection of new interventions for recurrent fallers. Each team received a 69 page manual, a videotape for staff training and other resources describing examples of case histories.

Data was gathered on process of care documentation, common falls, and physical restraint use rates.

The authors reported that several areas of documentation regarding assessment and management of falls improved significantly. Fall rates were not significantly different between the intervention and control nursing homes. The use of restraint techniques decreased substantially during the project period from 7.9% to 4.4% in the intervention nursing homes. This was a relative reduction of 44% but there also a decrease in the non-intervention/ control nursing homes from 7.0 to 4.9% (a relative reduction of 30%). Fall rates remained stable in the intervention nursing homes whereas fall rates increased 20% in the control nursing homes.

The authors concluded that implementation of the training was associated with significantly improved care process documentation with a non-changing stable fall rate during the study period but a substantial reduction in the use of physical restraint. In contrast, the fall rates increased in the control nursing homes.

In summary, there is no detail described on the actual profile of those attending the education intervention, nor mention of attrition rate. There is no clear evidence in regard to the teaching methods that allows comparison with other studies nor to gauge at what level on the IPE continuum these interventions may have been.

Weaver et al. (2010) reported on an evaluation study aimed at improving team work for operating room (OR staff). There were 29 professionals in the intervention group and 26 in the control group. The profile of each (interventions vs controls) was surgeons (3 vs 2), certified registered nurse anaesthetists (6 vs 5), nurses (3 vs 13) surgical technicians (3 vs 3), anaesthesiologists (12 vs 3) and physician assistants (2 vs 0). The intervention group participated in TeamSTEPPS training. This consisted of a four hours didactic session including interactive role paly. A detailed set of competencies was described within three main areas, communication, mutual support and situation monitoring. The control group received no training.

Data was gathered by observed changes in collaborative behaviour, which included frequency of team briefings in which information was shared amongst team members and how patient care was planned.

The authors reported that the intervention group engaged in significantly more team pre-case briefings after the TeamSTEPPS training (p < 0.001). There was also a significant increase in the proportion of information sharing (p < 0.001).

In terms of IPE although a set of high level competencies was stated it is difficult to infer the extent to which the methods allowed any level of IPE. There was a detailed breakdown of the different professionals and in addition their years in the current post.

Young et al. (2005) described a study evaluating the effects of a consumer-led innovation with the aim of improving the competencies of mental health practitioners working within communal health settings. The study was conducted at five large community health provider organisations in two Western states in the USA, Arizona and Colorado. The focus was involvement in a consumer-focused intervention with six main themes for the clinicians involved:

Scientific presentation on self-help
Structured dialogue
Rehabilitation readiness
Strategies for independence
Professional skills supporting self-help
Detailing

One organisation in each state received the intervention, which included an initial one day at each site with research presentations, structured questions, and small group work. The instructors visited each site for a further four days and three days in Arizona and Colorado respectively. In addition, there was a further 16 hours described as spent in meetings at various times with staff at the sites. The interventions spanned a 12-month period.

A total of 269 clinicians participated in the study with 151 in the intervention group and 118 in the control group. The profile of professionals in the intervention vs control were:

Clinician or therapist 72 vs 12

Residential staff 27 vs 43

Mental health worker 12 vs 30

Case manager 10 vs 16

Administrative support 14 vs 12

Nurse 10 vs 3

Psychiatrist 2 vs 0 (not all data were available for all participants)

Data were collected at base-line and at one year. The authors reported that the practitioners in the intervention group reported significantly higher scores in relation to the follow-up competencies of team work, holistic approach, education about care, rehabilitation methods and overall competency.

Detail of the professional profiles of the intervention and control groups are described. From the description of the education intervention there is no clear evidence to clarify the level of IPE strategies used.

Time Interrupted Series Studies (TIS)

Time interrupted series (TIS) studies collect data at multiple instances over time before and after the intervention (the 'interruption'). This allows the measurement of the effect of the intervention in contrast to the underlying secular trends (Ramsay et al. 2003). So, an advantage of the TIS design is that is allows for the statistical investigation of a range of potential biases including:

1 Secular trend – this is when the outcome may be increasing or decreasing over time. So if the observed outcomes were 'naturally' increasing before the intervention one could have wrongly attributed the observed effect to the intervention under study if for example, a before-and-after study was performed.

2 Cyclical or seasonal effects – the outcome may vary over a certain time period in a cyclical pattern

3 Duration of the intervention – the intervention may for example have an effect only in the first three months after it was introduced. In that scenario data collected on an annual basis would not detect the effect.

4 Random fluctuations – these can be brief fluctuations with no recognisable pattern that can bias outcomes.

5 Autocorrelation – this is the degree to which data collected close together in time are correlated with each other.

Hanbury et al. (2009) reported a time series study with the aim of evaluating the impact of a theory of planned behaviour (TPB) intervention on health professions adherence to national suicide prevention guidelines. In its simplest terms the TPB (Ajzen 1988) is used to study various behaviours and intentions. TPB states that intention, one the immediate determinants of behaviour, relies on three constructs; attitudes, subjective norms and perceived behavioural control. In turn, these direct constructs are influenced by the indirect constructs of behavioural, normative, and control beliefs respectively (see Chapter 2 for more on TPB).

The study was conducted in an NHS Trust in the West Midlands, UK. All community mental health professionals on the intervention site were invited to participate. The intervention was delivered to 49 participants. The intervention, an educational session, had three elements:

1 a presentation containing factual statements, statistics and graphs in support of the national guidelines;

2 a facilitated group discussion to ensure positive normative beliefs were emphasised; and

3 group work based on two real-life case studies; one describing a case where national guidelines were adhered to and a near miss was avoided and the second where guidelines weren't adhered to with a resulting negative outcome.

No professional or discipline breakdown of the participants is provided by the authors.

Data was collected via routine monthly audit adherence for 28 months pre intervention and 18 months post. Data from a control site were collected for a comparison. The authors reported that the intervention did not significantly increase adherence to the guidelines.

There are some key questions in regard to this study. The third phase of the intervention was small group work using a case-based type approach. Neither the duration nor specific objectives and teaching methods used are reported. The absence of detail in regard to the professional profile of the group may call into question how interprofessional the group was. This is perhaps not too surprising as the focus in the study was the use of TPB as a theory to underpin the intervention, while evaluation of an IPE intervention was not a stated objective.

Taylor et al. (2007) described a time series analysis with the aim of assessing the effects of an intervention on evidence-based diabetes care standards, work processes and patient outcomes. The setting was an inner-city primary care clinic in Nashville, Tennessee, USA.

The profile of the participants is not clearly described but reference is made to 'APN, support staff and administrators'.

The intervention was of eight hours duration and comprised of what was described as common components of crew resource management (CRM) including:

Task redistribution;

Standardised communication methods; and

Decision support tool (checklist) development.

Measures of 619 patients (e.g. blood sugar, blood pressure, low density lipoprotein) were taken on 160 pre-intervention and 122 post-intervention clinic days. The results showed improved compliance with microalbumin testing.

In the absence of detail in regard to the professional profile and numerical balance of the participants it is difficult to judge the extent of a real inter-professional approach. The teaching methods are not clearly described and so again it is difficult to make a judgement as to where this educational intervention lay on the IPE continuum.

Summary of Reeves et al. (2013) Review

In this Cochrane Review the inclusion criteria were extremely broad and three types of study were included, RCT, CBA and TIS. This process identified a number of studies with limited evidence of the effectiveness of IPE teaching or learning strategies per se. In some studies the profile of learners was not described in detail and frequently the educational methodologies used do not allow consideration of the extent of true IPE undertaken.

Reeves et al. (2017) Review

Reeves et al. (2017) undertook a further Cochrane review but used different inclusion and exclusion criteria as below:
- Only considered individual or cluster randomised studies; and
- Participants included any health and or social care professionals.
  The definition of the educational intervention included was:

> *Practice based intervention with the explicit objective of improving collaboration between two or more health or social care professionals*
>
> (Reeves et al. 2017, p. 8)

Outcome measures included were:

1 Primary outcomes … patient health outcomes; clinical process or efficiency outcomes.
2 Secondary outcomes … collaborative behaviour – objective or self-reported outcomes, using a validated instrument.

The protocol specifically excluded interprofessional learning and interprofessional education as a secondary outcome.

As a result of the different focus of this review compared to 2013 further papers were considered and a selection are detailed and critiqued below.

Black et al. (2013) described a cluster randomised trial to test the effectiveness of an intervention on the quality of care for patients with diabetes, ischaemic heart disease or /hypertension. The location was urban and rural New South Wales, Victoria and the Australian Capital Territory.

The participants were staff in 60 general practices that were randomised to the educational intervention immediately or after 12 months. The professional profile included General Practitioners (GPs), nurses, and administrative staff but excluded allied health professionals. The numerical break down of each group is not described.

The intervention was based on 11 elements from previous work that are known to contribute to enhanced teamwork for chronic conditions;

Structured appointment systems
Patient disease registers
Recall and reminders
Patient education
Planned care
Practice-based linkages
Roles, responsibilities and job descriptions
Communication and meetings
Practice billing
Record keeping
Quality

The intervention was an education session of one to two hours with GP and non-GP staff. This was followed by three one-hour practice visits with the named practice study lead and other staff. Resource manuals and workbooks for each of the 11 elements were provided to all participants. During the follow up visits each practice team identified one of the 11 elements as a priority for the team to focus on.

Assessment measurements were taken at 12 months post intervention. All staff were asked to complete the chronic care team profile (CCTP) that measures multidisciplinary teamwork structures and functions.

Patients completed the patient assessment of chronic illness care (PACIC) (final sample n = 1853 patients) questionnaire. This is a 20-item questionnaire where patients rate quality of care on a five-point Likert scale.

The results showed that the intervention practice teams had a greater increase in team profile scores compared to controls indicating an increased role for non-medical staff in patient management. There was no significant difference in patient-reported quality of care between the intervention and control teams.

The authors concluded that their results suggested that more time was required for organisational change to occur.

With this study a detailed profile of the participating professionals was not described and with the intervention it was difficult to compare across other similar studies.

Calland et al. (2011) reported a randomised trial to test the effectiveness of procedural checklists for surgical teams during laparoscopic cholecystectomies. The location was the Department of Surgery, University of Virginia School of Medicine, USA.

The participants were 10 general surgery attending physicians who volunteered to undertake the study. There were 23 patients in the intervention group and 18 in the control.

The surgeons were randomised to the intervention (n = 5), which comprised basic team training and the use of a perioperative checklist. The control group (n = 5) performed standard cholecystectomies. All procedures were videotaped and scored by trained reviewers, for the presence of safety critical behaviours.

There were no differences in any measures of patient outcomes between the two groups. The intervention cases were significantly more likely to involve positive safety-related team behaviours such as explicit discussions of roles and responsibilities, contingency planning, equipment checks and postoperative debriefings.

In this study, although there is mention of 'a briefing with introductions of all team members' there appears to be just one profession as the participants. The intervention comprised the provision of instructions on how to use the check list and hence does not map to any previously described IPE approach.

Cheater et al. (2005) described a randomised trial of 22 multi-disciplinary teams (MDTs) to assess the impact of an intervention to promote a MD approach to audit. The MDTs were based in secondary care, in five acute hospital sites in the East Midlands, UK.

The study teams comprised a mix of specialities including surgery, medicine, accident and emergency, nephrology, respiratory medicine, obstetrics and gynaecology, orthopaedics, rheumatology and rehabilitation, elderly care, and general psychiatry. There were 11 intervention (n = 77) and 11 control teams (n = 64) (Table 3.1).

Table 3.1 The study teams.

Intervention teams	Control teams
Nurses 29 (38%)	25 (39%)
Doctors 16 (21%)	16 (25%)
PAMs[a] 12 (16%)	13 (20%)
SSS[b] 9 (12%)	6 (9%)
Managers 8 (10%)[c]	4 (6%)

[a] PAMs = professions allied to medicine, pharmacist, social worker, physiotherapist
[b] SSS = service support staff
[c] not all data were available for all participants

The intervention comprised five facilitated meetings over a six-month period. Activities were described as supporting MDTs to undertake an audit. The intervention teams were required to undertake an audit and submit a report as a part of the intervention. The control teams were also required to submit an audit and they had access to the usual support tools.

Knowledge, skills and attitudes of participants were measured immediately post-intervention and at four months. Collaborative behaviour was measured via self-reporting using a version of the Collaborative Practice Scales (CPS; Weiss and Davis 1985). In addition, two of the intervention meetings were videoed and rated by one researcher for small-group interaction.

Self-reported knowledge and skills were significantly improved immediately post and four months post-intervention. Attitude to audit was significantly improved immediately post-intervention only. There was a statistically significant improvement in self-reported and observed collaborative behaviour. The authors speculate that the improved collaborative behaviour may be due to increased assertive behaviour of the nurses as measured via the CPS. Participation in the intervention was associated with increased audit activity with 9 of the 11 teams reporting improvement in care and 7 completing an audit cycle.

In this study the detail of the professionals involved reflect an appropriate multiprofessional balance but the intervention was focused on enhancing audit and the detail provided makes it difficult to compare the teaching strategies with other studies.

Curley et al. (1998) reported a randomised controlled firm trial of the effect of interdisciplinary rounds on patient outcomes. The location was at the MetroHealth Medical Centre, USA and involved six acute medical wards. Patients were randomly assigned to either the three intervention (n = 567 patients) or the control wards (n = 535 patients).

Participants involved interns and residents in medicine, staff nurses, nursing supervisors, respirologists, pharmacists, nutritionists and social workers. Details of the participants are not provided.

The intervention consisted of daily interdisciplinary rounds over a six-month period. The control teams received no additional intervention and followed usual pre-existing firm systems and processes.

The outcome measures for each patient included LOS, total hospital charges, provider satisfaction and ancillary staff efficiency. The key finding was that the mean LOS for the intervention group was significantly less that of the control, 5.46 vs 6.06 days (p = 0.002). There was a similar significant reduction in total charges for the two groups.

The staff were asked to complete a survey designed to evaluate:
1 the perceived teaching value of rounds
2 the efficiency of rounds
3 the interdisciplinary communication on the ward
Nineteen providers of the traditional rounds (the control) and 21 in the intervention group completed surveys. There were statistically significant higher scores in the intervention group for all three measures (p < 0.006 for each).

This study does not provide detail on the professionals involved and the description of the intervention does not allow comparison or bench marking to recognised IPE type approaches.

Deneckere et al. (2013) reported a cluster RCT evaluating the impact of care pathways intervention on interprofessional team working in acute hospital settings in Belgium. The aim was to evaluate whether the implementation of care pathways (CPs) improved teamwork in acute hospital settings.

The patient groups were those with proximal fracture of the femur (PFF) and exacerbation of chronic obstructive pulmonary disease (COPD). Seventeen intervention clinical teams were compared to 13 controls. There were 346 participants in the intervention group versus 235 in the control.

The professional breakdown was stated as:
Medical doctors 75 (13%)
Head nurses 33 (6%)
Nurses 379 (65%)
Allied health professions 94 (16%)

The intervention had three elements.
1 A pre-study evaluation of each team's performance with a detailed report provided to each team.
2 Each team received a set of evidence-based key interventions (KIs) relevant to the two disease groups under study. These were delivered via a workshop.
3 Each team was trained in care pathway.

The intervention teams showed better interprofessional teamwork, higher levels of organised care, higher leadership structures, higher use of guidelines and increased frequency of team meetings. These were assessed via structured questionnaires. They also reported a lower risk of burnout.

The authors concluded that CP interventions lead to improved teamwork, increased organisational levels of care processes, and decreased the risk of burnout for health care teams in acute hospital settings.

Schmidt et al. (1998) reported a randomised trial of 33 nursing homes with the aim of testing the effects of monthly, facilitated MD rounds on the quality and quantity of psychotropic drug prescribing. The location was from across regions in Sweden.

There were 15 intervention (n = 626 residents) and 18 control homes (n = 1228 residents), representing 5% of all homes in Sweden.

The outcome measures used were the number and type of drugs prescribed before and after the invention.

The intervention lasted over a 12-month period with a selected pharmacist spending one day a week in the experimental homes and helping to organise regular MDT meetings. Sessions focused on reviewing drug usage of individual residents and all staff were encouraged to participate.

There is reference to physicians, pharmacists, staff nurses and nursing assistants but a detailed profile of the participants was not provided.

The results show that after the 12-month intervention there was a significant decrease in use of psychotics (−19%), benzodiazepine hypnotics (−37%), and anti-depressants (−59%). The authors' summary is that improved team work can improve prescribing.

As neither the details of the participants nor the teaching strategies used were described it is difficult to compare across to other studies or to replicate.

Wild et al. (2004) described a randomised trial to evaluate the impact of daily interdisciplinary rounds (IRs) on patient outcome measures. The trial was carried out in an inpatient telemetry ward in a community hospital in Derby, Connecticut, USA. Forty-two patients were randomised to the intervention team and 42 to the control team, involving pre-existing standard care.

The participants were resident physicians, nurses, a case manager, pharmacist, dietician and physical therapist. Details of the participants were not described. The intervention consisted of daily interdisciplinary rounds when all staff met to discuss patients and to address any issues delaying discharge.

The main outcome measure was LOS. The staff involved in the intervention completed a questionnaire (response rate 80%) rating improvement in communication and optimised timing of discharge.

The authors report that there was no statistically significant difference in LOS between the two groups of patients. It is reported that staff generally felt very positive about the IRs. No further detail is provided.

This study involved a small clinical team and small sample size of patients and hence these factors could be argued to account for the observed no difference between the two groups.

Wilson et al. (2004) described a RCT testing the effectiveness of multi-disciplinary case conferencing using audio-visual compared with telephone only communication.

The location was two hospitals, Campbelltown and Camden, New South Wales, Australia. Fifty patients were randomly assigned to either the audio-visual or telephone multi-disciplinary case conferencing. The participants were 2 medical staff specialists, 2 medical registrars, 15 nurses, 1 speech pathologist, 2 occupational therapists, 1 social worker and 6 medical students (total number = 29). The intervention was either video or telephone case conferencing. There was no educational intervention described.

Outcome measures included number of conference sessions per patient, average length of conference, length of treatment, and number of occasions of service. The mean number of case conferences for the audiovisual group was less and had a shorter length of treatment (6 vs 10 days) for the intervention vs control. The introduction of the video-link was rated highly by the team members in the intervention group.

This study set out to compare telephone versus videoconferencing in a MDT setting. There was no educational intervention.

Broader Benefits of IPE for Stakeholders

There are arguments supporting the case for IPE to provide a range of benefits for the learner(s), employers and education organisations that deliver the teaching, universities, the NHS and postgraduate deaneries.

Shakman et al. (2013) explored the potential benefits for each of these stakeholders summarised in Table 3.2.

It is useful to reflect on one of these points in the table in some more detail: the opportunity that IPE can afford for the development of collaborative competencies.

Some of these include (Barr 2005):

Describe one's roles and responsibilities clearly to other professions.

Recognise the constraints and limits of one's own role and competencies.

Recognise the needs of patients in the wider context, outside of one's responsibilities.

Table 3.2 Summary of finding reported by Shakman et al. (2013).

1. Employers
Improved communication between heath professionals
Increased morale and efficiency
A breakdown of potentially destructive professional silos
2. Learners
Improves leaners' understanding of other professional roles
Exposure to positive interprofessional role models
Facilitates development of collaborative competencies
3. Training providers (universities, health organisations)
Cost effectiveness
Developing the skills to work in MDTs
Bring students (if in HEI setting) together from different degrees/programmes
Staff can be exposed to new ideas, work with a wider diversity of colleagues
Improved networking/collaboration between departments

Source Adapted from Shakman, L., Renu, G. and Obeidat, A. (2013). Inter professional education in health care. *International Journal of Nursing Education* 5 (1): 86–91.

Respect the roles and responsibilities of others.

Tolerate differences in other professions.

Develop and enhance interdependent relations with other professions.

Chapter Summary

A criticism of the studies explored in this chapter is that the specific teaching strategies used are not described. This makes it difficult to ascertain what level if any the interventions were at. A regular theme is team training which has a multitude of definitions (see Chapter 2). Other specific approaches used, including the PRECEDE/PROCEED and the Theory of Planned Behaviour do not readily sit or align with the published work on 'pure' IPE.

So, the question remains as to what aspects of IPE are effective. The studies reported here, as just examples, show a wide and diverse range of outcomes, from improved blood glucose control (Janson et al. 2009) to improved confidence in asking about domestic violence (Thompson et al. 2000b). However, some studies showed no statistically significant effects of IPE-type education interventions. The heterogeneity of the educational interventions makes it difficult to draw general conclusions of the effects of particular aspects of the IPE experience.

The question is in what circumstances can this innovative group of teaching strategies be best used? Harden provided a three-dimension model almost 20 years ago and although it has limited use there has been no practical model.

Barr's dimensions do provide a guide for learners and designers/providers of IPE. Xyrichis et al. (2017) described a framework (see Chapter 6). This may turn out to be a practical tool for researchers and educators to use to identify at what level their education interventions lie. The following questions need to asked and answered within the methodology for any study seeking to answer the 'effectiveness question' for IPE.

1 In what context is the IPE is to be used?
2 What are the expected learning objectives?
3 Which specific teaching strategies along the IPE continuum are to used? Going forward it is essential that Xyrichis et al.'s InterPACT (2017) is tested to evaluate its effectiveness as a practical tool.
4 At what level are we seeking to show impact, at an individual patient level, health population level, staff attitude or team working ability?

Any further research need to address the following:

1 Larger sample sizes;
2 More appropriate control groups;
3 Explicit focus on specific aspects of IPE. This is key and is a frequent 'flaw' in published work. It is essential that researchers make explicit the exact teaching methods used and a measure of the degree or extent of IPE, with a clear description of the professional/disciplinary profile of the participants.
4 Rigorous randomisation procedures;
5 Allocation concealment;
6 More sophisticated outcome measures such as changes in health care processes, individual and population health outcomes with studies aimed at exploring compliance with the Triple Aim.

References

Ajzen, I. (1988). *Attitudes, Personality, and Behavior*. Chicago: Dorsey Press.

Barceló, A., Cafiero, E., de Boer, M. et al. (2010). Using collaborative learning to improve diabetes care and outcomes: The VIDA project. *Primary Care Diabetes* 4 (3): 145–153.

Barr, H. (1996). Ends and means in interprofessional education: towards a typology. *Education for Health* 9 (3): 341–352.

Barr, H. (2005). *Interprofessional Education. Today, Yesterday and Tomorrow. A Review*. London: The UK Centre for the Advancement in Interprofessional Education.

Black, D.A., Taggart, J., Jayasinghe, U.W. et al. (2013). The Teamwork Study: enhancing the role of non-GP staff in chronic disease management in general practice. *Australian Journal of Primary Health* 19 (3): 184–189.

Brown, J.B., Boles, M., Mullooly, J.P. et al. (1999). Effect of clinician communication skills training on patient satisfaction: a randomised controlled trial. *Annals of Internal Medicine* 131 (11): 822–829.

Calland, J.F., Turrentine, F.E., Guerlain, S. et al. (2011). The surgical safety checklist: lessons learned during implementation. *The American Surgeon* 77 (9): 1131–1137.

Campbell, J.C., Coben, J.H., McLoughlin, E. et al. (2001). An evaluation of a system –change training model to improve emergency department response to battered women. *Academic Emergency Medicine* 8 (20): 131–138.

Cheater, F.M., Hearnshaw, H., Baker, R. et al. (2005). Can a facilitated programme promote effective multidisciplinary audit in secondary care teams? An exploratory trial. *International Journal of Nursing Studies* 42: 779–791.

Curley, C., McEachern, J.E., and Speroff, T. (1998). A firm trial of interdisciplinary rounds on the inpatient medical wards. *Medical Care* 36 (8): AS4–AS12.

Deneckere, S., Euwema, M., Lodewijckx, C. et al. (2013). Better interprofessional teamwork., higher level of organized care, and lower risk of burnout in acute health care teams using care pathways: a cluster randomized controlled trial. *Medical Care* 51 (1): 99–107.

Hanbury, A., Wallace, L., and Clarke, M. (2009). Use of a time series design to test effectiveness of a theory-based intervention targeting adherence of health professionals to a clinical guideline. *British Journal of Health Psychology* 14 (Pt 3): 505–518.

Harden, R.M. (2000). The integration ladder: a tool for curriculum planning. *Medical Education* 34: 551–557.

Harden, R.M., Sowden, S., and Dunn, W.R. (1984). Educational strategies in curriculum development: the SPICES model. *Medical Education* 18: 284–297.

Helitzer, D.L., LaNoue, M., Wilson, B. et al. (2011). A randomized controlled trial of communication training with primary care providers to improve patient-centeredness and health risk communication. *Patient Education and Counseling* 82 (1): 21–29. https://doi.org/10.1016/j.pec.2010.01.021.

Janson, S.l., Cooke, M., McGrath, K.W. et al. (2009). Improving chronic care of Type 2 diabetes using teams of interprofessional learners. *Academic Medicine* 84: 1540–1548.

Lichstein, K.L., Riedel, B.W., and Grieve, R. (1994). Fair tests of clinical trials: a treatment implementation model. *Advances in Behaviour Research Therapy* 16: 1–29.

Locke, A., Evangelista, J., Langford, V. et al. (2001). *MedTeams Emergency Team Coordination Course*. Andover, MA: Dynamics Research Corporation.

Morey, J.C., Simon, R., Jay, G.D. et al. (2002). Error reduction and performance improvement in the emergency department through formal teamwork training: evaluation results of the MedTeams project. *Health Service Research* 37 (6): 1553–1581.

Nielsen, P.E., Goldman, M.D., Mann, S. et al. (2007). Effects of teamwork training on adverse outcomes and process of care in labor and delivery. *Obstetrics and Gynecology* 109 (1): 48–55.

Ramsay, C.R., Matowe, L., Grilli, R. et al. (2003). Interrupted time series designs in health technology assessment; lessons from two systematic reviews of behaviour change strategies. *International Journal of Technology Assessment in Health Care* 19 (4): 613–623.

Rask, K., Parmelee, P.A., Taylor, J. et al. (2007). Implementation and evaluation of a nursing home fall management program. *Journal of the American Geriatrics Society* 55: 342–349.

Reeves, S., Pelone, F., Harrison, R. et al. (2017). Interprofessional collaboration to improve professional practice and healthcare outcomes. *The Cochrane Database of Systematic Reviews* 6: CD000072.

Reeves, S., Perrier, L., Goldman, J. et al. (2013). Interprofessional education: effects on professional practice and healthcare outcomes (update). *The Cochrane Database of Systematic Reviews* 3: CD002213.

Risser, D.T., Rice, M.L., Salisbury, R. et al. (1999). The potential for improved teamwork to reduce medical errors in the emergency department. *Annals of Emergency Medicine* 34 (3): 373–383.

Schmidt, I., Claesson, C.B., Westerholm, B. et al. (1998). The impact of regular multidisciplinary team interventions on psychotropic prescribing in Swedish nursing homes. *Journal of the American Geriatrics Society* 46: 77–82.

Shakman, L., Renu, G., and Obeidat, A. (2013). Inter professional education in health care. *International Journal of Nursing Education* 5 (1): 86–91.

Stolberg, H.O., Norman, G., and Trop, I. (2004). Fundaments of clinical research for radiologists. *American Journal of Roentgenology* 183 (6): 1539–1544.

Strasser, D.C., Falconer, J.A., Stevens, A.B. et al. (2008). Team training and stroke rehabilitation outcomes: a cluster randomized trial. *Archives of Physical Medicine Rehabilitation* 89: 10–15.

Taylor, C.R., Hepworth, J.T., Buerhaus, P.I. et al. (2007). Effect of crew resource management on diabetes care and patient outcomes in an inner-city primary care clinic. *Quality and Safety in Health Care* 16: 244–247.

Thompson, C., Kinmonth, A.L., Stevens, L. et al. (2000a). Effects of clinical guidelines and practice-based education on detection and outcome of depression in primary care: Hampshire depression project randomised controlled trial. *Lancet* 355: 185–191.

Thompson, R.S., Meyer, B.A., and Smith-DiJulio, K. et al. (1998). A training program to improve domestic violence identification and management in primary care: preliminary results. *Violence and Victims* 13 (4): 395–410.

Thompson, R.S., Rivara, F.P., Thompson, D.C. et al. (2000b). Identification and management of domestic violence a randomized trial. *American Journal of Preventative Medicine* 19 (4): 253–263.

Wahlstrom, O. and Sanden, I. (1998). Multiprofessional training at Linköping University; early experiences. *Education for Health* 11: 225–231.

Weaver, S.J., Rosen, M.A., DiazGranados, D. et al. (2010). Does teamwork improve performance in the operating room? A multilevel evaluation. *The Joint Commission Journal on Quality and Patient Safety* 36 (3): 133–142.

Weiss, S.L. and Davis, P.H. (1985). Validity and reliability of the collaborative practice scales. *Nursing Research* 34: 299–302.

Wild, D., Nawaz, H., Chan, W. et al. (2004). Effects of interdisciplinary rounds on length of stay in a telemetry unit. *Journal of Public Health Management Practice* 10 (1): 63–69.

Wilson, S.F., Marks, R., Collins, N. et al. (2004). Benefits of multidisciplinary case conferencing using audiovisual compared with telephone communication: a randomized controlled trial. *Journal of Telemedicine and Telecare* 10 (6): 351–354.

Xyrichis, A., Reeves, S., and Zwarenstein, M. (2017). Examining the nature of interprofessional practice: an initial framework validation and creation of the Interprofessional Activity Classification Tool (InterPACT). *Journal of Interprofessional Care* https://doi.org/10.1080/13561820.2017.1408576.

Young, A.S., Chinman, M., Forquer, S.L. et al. (2005). Use of a consumer-led intervention to improve provider competencies. *Psychiatric Services* 56: 967–975.

Zigmond, A.S. and Snaith, R.P. (1983). The hospital anxiety and depression rating scale. *Acta Psychiatrica Scandinavica* 67: 361–370.

Chapter 4 **Design Principles for Interprofessional Education**

Who is this chapter for? It is aimed at:
1 those currently responsible for the design of Interprofessional Education (IPE) learning
2 learners currently on a course/programme of learning with elements of IPE
3 institutions that commission IPE training/education or are considering doing so

Introduction

This chapter will describe the principles underpinning the successful delivery of IPE and highlight the barriers to this and offer solutions.

Health care in the twenty-first century is increasingly delivered by multidisciplinary teams and with the recognition that integrated care provides patients with higher quality service, the role of IPE is increasingly important. There are a number of terms used interchangeably, multiprofessional, interprofessional and poly professional. One of the barriers to the more widespread adoption of IPE has been lack of clarity around these definitions and how each is implemented (see Chapter 2 for definitions).

Before exploring specific design principles and their practical application it is useful to consider just where your current or proposed IPE-type course or programme sits within accepted models of IPE. Harden's ladder (2000) is useful as a starting point to help to gauge where your teaching or learning sits. This will ultimately help shape and determine the design and details of teaching methods used. Harden described IPE as having three dimensions:
1 the context;
2 the learning objectives; and
3 the specific approach that will be used to deliver the learning, that is, which teaching strategies across a continuum will be used that best fit the context and the expected objectives.

How to Succeed at Interprofessional Education, First Edition. Peter Donnelly.
© 2019 John Wiley & Sons Ltd. Published 2019 by John Wiley & Sons Ltd.

In regard to this third dimension, the particular approaches that can be used lie along a continuum with isolation (uniprofessional [UP]) at one end to trans-disciplinary ('transprofessional') at the other. Harden described these as 11 steps in multiprofessional education.

Harden's (2000) 11 steps are:

1 Isolation
2 Awareness
3 Harmonisation
4 Nesting
5 Temporal co-ordination
6 Sharing
7 Correlation
8 Complementary
9 Multi-disciplinary
10 Inter-disciplinary
11 Trans-disciplinary

Each of these levels is a description essentially based on the level of collaboration. There is a balance between integration and solely subject based with the latter being the focus up to and including the nesting step on the ladder. It must be remembered that each is a reasonable and appropriate teaching approach depending on the specific aims and objectives of the course or programme. See Chapter 3 for more detail.

Using Harden's ladder one can get a sense of where your programme lies or where it could lie. This can then be used as a baseline for design and for considering what steps you might want to take to move the learning from say nesting to the next level or decide that, for your learners, nesting is an appropriate strategy at this point.

In reality, these points along the continuum are not static and in a professional career your learners are likely to have exposure to learning experiences using most if not all of these steps. There is an argument for a planned approach to career development starting with UP at the beginning to engender a sense of identity and equip learners with basic profession-specific skills and then in a programmed fashion expose them to increasing IPE cycles of learning.

Although Harden's proposed ladder is a useful starting point, it does not provide clarity for researchers. A practical tool is needed. Further work has been undertaken by Reeves et al. (2011) to improve the conceptual clarity of IP interventions. Xyrichis et al. (2017) who considered this issue against a background of the need to clarify definitions and provide a practical framework, described the Interprofessional Activity Classification Tool (InterPACT). These will be described in detail in Chapter 6.

General Education Principles

There are general educational principles that apply across any modality and along all the points in Harden's continuum. For completeness, some of these will be explored. These will be addressed under the following headings;

1 Learning Needs Analysis
2 Aims
3 Learning outcomes
4 Lesson plans
5 Feedback

Learning Needs Analysis

Before embarking on any learning strategy, it is essential to be aware of individual's and the group's learning needs. This must take into account prior learning and any subsequent gaps in knowledge or skills. The new learning can then be targeted to meeting these needs.

The concept of learning needs analysis comes from the theory of adult learning and is the process by which the learner, through reflection, identifies gaps in knowledge or skills. Knowledge and understanding of these gaps then helps inform the generation of an action plan (Knowles et al. 2011). This self-assessment process, underpinned by the process of reflection is the first step in any adult learning and is pivotal in any continuing professional development.

It is important to distinguish between perceived and true learning needs (Laxdal 1982). There is an argument that true learning needs are personal, owned and identified by the individual. Identification of learning needs comes through reflection, both internal and external. The external element has been described as informed self-assessment (Sargeant et al. 2010) informed through reference to external standards such as those set out by the individual's regulator.

However, when such external benchmarking is not available, or is not referred to, then the process of self-assessment of perceived needs becomes increasingly subjective. With this scenario, there is a risk that solely self-assessed perceived needs may not necessarily reflect all that is required.

In comparison, true learning needs are objectively generated by external independent assessment of a learner's performance against an agreed standard. This process involves triangulation of information from a range of sources, methods and collection strategies (Lockyer 1998). The sources can include peers, educational supervisors, mentors and patients. There are risks with this approach, since if a learner perceives that learning is imposed on them there is likely to be less of a feeling of ownership, which increases the likelihood of disengagement.

	Learning Needs Known to Learner	Learning Needs Unknown to Learner
Learning Needs Known to Tutor	1 Open	2 Blind
Learning Needs Unknown to Tutor	3 Hidden	4 Unknown

Figure 4.1 The Johari window adapted for use in an educational setting. (Adapted from Luft, J. and Ingham, H. [1950]. The Johari window, a graphic model of interpersonal awareness. *Proceedings of the Western Training Laboratory in Group Development.* Los Angeles: UCLA).

A useful tool to explore one's perceived and true learning needs is the Johari window, as shown in Figure 4.1 (Luft and Ingham 1950). The Johari window is a simple psychological tool, visually represented as four windows, that facilities personal self-awareness. It has since been revised and adapted for use in a wide range of scenarios and is particularly useful in education/training settings.

In the context of learning needs, panes one and three reflect the learner's awareness of their own learning needs and as such represent the individual's perceived learning needs. In pane one, these are also known by the trainer or teacher. However in pane three, these needs are only known to the learner. Panes two and four reflect learning needs that the learners themselves do not acknowledge or have insight to. In pane two the learning needs are unknown by the individual but known to others. So, pane four reflects the scenario whereby neither the learner nor trainer is aware of learning needs, though these exist. Therefore, panes two and four represent the true learning needs.

Reflective Cycles and Action Plans
As an adult learner (Knowles 1980) and clinician, reflection is key to the learning process. In fact, reflection is a basic tool used by humans to make sense of complex or ambiguous situations and to learn from these experiences.

There are many definitions of reflection. As just one example Moon (1999) states:

a form of mental processing with a purpose and/or anticipated outcome that is applied to relatively complex or unstructured ideas for which there is not an obvious solution.

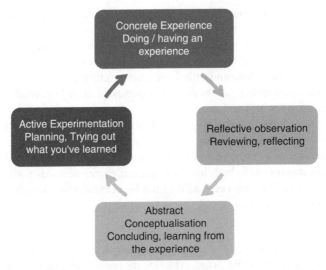

Figure 4.2 Kolb's learning cycle. (Adapted from Kolb, DA. [1984]. *Experiential Learning: Experience as a Source of Learning and Development.* New Jersey: Prentice Hall).

The seminal work of Schön (1983) embedded the important concept of the reflective practitioner and described two types of reflection. First reflection-in-action that occurs at the time of the 'incident' and refection-on-action, a process that occurs sometime after the event. Both of these are iterative processes and can lead to learning from one experience being incorporated into future 'knowing-in-action'.

Another definition of reflection is offered by Boyd and Fales (1983):

> *the process of internally examining and exploring an issue of concern, triggered by an experience, which creates and clarifies meaning in terms of self, and which results in a changed conceptual perspective.*

Kolb (1984) described a four-stage model of reflective practice based on experiential learning that is applicable for learning in clinical practice. This is shown in Figure 4.2.

Kolb's cycle describes that the experience of an event in itself is not enough to promote learning. In addition, the learner must reflect on their experiences and make links between theory and action in order to truly promote learning. However, in order to close the 'learning gap' between the learner's current performance and expected competency, an action plan must be created to address this. The SMART approach is a widely used method for generating a well-structured and meaningful action plan.

Specific: Learning outcomes need to be clearly defined and easily communicated.

Measurable: What is expected at the end of the learning must be easily measured so that the learner can assess if they have been successful.

Achievable: It is vital that any objectives set are realistic and achievable within the time frame and with the resources available.

Relevant: The learning must be perceived as relevant to the learner otherwise barriers to learning will develop.

Timely: each objective must be given a clear time line for achievement and if necessary interim milestones can help assessment of progress.

In summary, identifying learning needs is not a straight-forward task and involves incorporating both learner-generated perceived needs with more objective true learning needs as directed by external sources such as the learner's trainer/teacher.

Aims

As a general principle the starting point in any learning experience is the learning outcomes (LOs). Before exploring the learning outcomes it is essential to understand the difference between LOs and aims.

An aim of a course or programme is essentially a broad statement of the purpose of the experience. This is a high-level statement and is written in general terms. An example of an IPE course for resuscitation training for nurses, doctors and technicians could be …

1 This training is designed to equip you with the skills and understanding to work effectively as part of a resuscitation team.

2 During the course the key elements of accredited resuscitation, using Resuscitation Council (UK) agreed protocols will be explored.

3 The course is designed to help you understand more fully the roles and responsibilities of all professionals and disciplines in the resuscitation team.

Learning Outcomes

In any learning it is vital for the teacher and learners to be clear what is expected of the learners. This applies equally to IPE. A systematic approach to writing learning outcomes was introduced as a way to express the type and depth of learning an assessment was supposed to measure. They can be seen as the 'specific, observable, and measurable' outcomes learners are expected to demonstrate after receiving instruction (Waller 1962).

Bloom's Taxonomy of Learning is the framework upon which this is based (Krathwohl 2002). This framework divides learning into three domains each with a hierarchy of six levels indicating the depth of learning to be demonstrated. The domains are:

Cognitive

Affective

Psychomotor

Table 4.1 Bloom's levels within the cognitive domain and examples of action verbs.

Bloom's levels within the cognitive domain	Example of action verbs
Knowledge	remembering information
Comprehension	being able to explain the information
Application	using the information in new ways
Analysis	to be able to identify different elements within it
Synthesis	use the information to form alternative solutions
Evaluation	challenge or defend ideas or concepts

Making the outcomes explicit helps to ensure that the assessments used actually assess these outcomes. Once we are clear about what our assessment criteria will be we can determine exactly what instructional material and activities the learner will need to be able to satisfy the assessment criteria.

Learning outcomes also serve a key role for learners enabling them to be proactive and self-directed, not just using whatever instructional material you provide but in addition access their own resources. This allows learners to cater for their own learning styles.

It is important to write out specific LOs for any learning be it a half-day or full three-year taught programme. Focusing on the cognitive domain (knowledge) Bloom described six levels (see Table 4.1).

With each of these levels, there are different action verbs used in writing the LOs. These are vital as they will dictate the resources, the teaching methods and the assessment methods used in the learning.

Table 4.2 shows each of the levels, a simple definition, examples of action verbs and example LOs for a multiprofessional resuscitation training programme.

Table 4.3 gives an example of a lesson plan.

Check list for writing LOs

Does each outcome start with an action verb?
Does it describe an outcome?
One action verb per outcome
Vary the action verbs
Do not use vague verbs such as 'understand' … be specific
LOs have to be at the right level
All LOs must be measurable
Can you easily collect data for each outcome?
Each LO must refer to the learner not what the tutor/trainer does
Do the LOs meet the aims of the learning?

Table 4.2 Examples of learning outcomes for a session of interprofessional resuscitation training.

Level	Definition	Action verbs	Sample learning outcome
Level 1. Remember	Learners show memory of new material by recalling facts, definitions, and basic concepts.	Recall, relate, quote, reproduce, list, name, define, select, describe, copy, identify	By the end of the training learners will be able to list the reversible causes of cardiac arrest.
Level 2. Understand	Learners demonstrate understanding of facts and ideas by summarising, classifying, comparing and explaining the key ideas.	Compare, explain, outline, summarise, select, paraphrase, differentiate, show, describe, ask, group, explain	By the end … learners will be able to differentiate between shockable and non-shockable rhythms.
Level 3. Apply	Learners solve problems by apply new knowledge, and skills in a different way.	Calculate, apply, solve, use, develop, make use of, plan, organise, predict, illustrate	Learners will be able to plan a co-ordinated approach to cardiac arrest.
Level 4. Analyse	Learners are able to breakdown information by identifying causes, relationships. They can make inferences and identify evidence to support generalisations.	Design, generate, modify, assess, compare, choose, prioritise, select, decide, award, explain, evaluate, judge, interpret	Learners will be able to select the appropriate air way device for different circumstances.
Level 5. Evaluate	Learners can weigh the information available and make judgements.	Modify, generate, decide, judge, measure, recommend, interpret, criticise, agree, create, formulate, rate, select	Learners will be able to judge when blood sampling is appropriate and prioritise interventions.
Level 6. Create	Learners are able to view information in a different way and generate new solutions.	Adapt, modify, invent, solve, hypothesise, collect, devise, design, construct, combine, plan, propose	Learners will be able design and adapt an algorithm for all cardiac crisis.

Table 4.3 Example of a lesson plan.

Topic/Title
The Mental Capacity Act 2005–the basics: an introduction
Aim of lesson
All participants will have a basic understanding of the five statutory principles of the Mental Capacity Act (MCA) and how they might apply in the context of their different working environments and a level of understanding of the effect on others and the need to work together.
Position of session/lesson in wider curriculum
This is a one off (three-hour) session at the request of local NHS and social services. There are currently no plans for any further sessions but there is clearly a need to build on this in the future.
Profile of learners
Mixture of social workers, care assistants (private and social services), GPs, mental health nurses
Learning outcomes
All leaners will:
1 Be able to recall the five key principles of the MCA
2 Understand that capacity is decision specific
3 Understand the role of the Court of Protection
4 Know how to contact their local Mental Capacity Advocates
(these are all at level 1)
Assumed prior knowledge/skills
A survey was sent to all expected participants (supplied by NHS and the Local Authority). All were asked about their prior training experience of the MCA. There was a range of prior knowledge but the majority of learners stated that they had little or no understanding (need to pitch level at this group but take into account those with some prior knowledge).
Resources needed
Power point (with audience response software)
Post it notes
Assessment
Assessment of learners:
For this, the Audience response system will be used throughout the session to ask basic questions mapped to the LOs.
Considering this is a three hour session as a one off I will use a simple online survey to measure learners' initial reaction to the session (pitched at Kirkpatrick's level 1).
Addressing all learners' needs
With a wide range of professionals/discipline groups which is likely to require a range of different leaning styles. Need to recognise VARK.
Information technology
Powerpoint
Email presentation
Mail draft FAQs to all and use to edit
Any learners with specific needs?
This was asked of all on the e-mail list prior to the session in initial survey and none declared

(Continued)

Table 4.3 (Continued)

Time	Teacher activity/content	Learner activity	resources
2.00	Introduction State aim of the session Ask each what they want to get out of the session		
	Split learners into pairs – buzz group	Discussion with peer then share with the wider group	Cabaret style tables
2.15	PowerPoint with 5 key principles of MCA 10 slides in total	Watch and listen	
2.45	Ask how might the first principle impact on your day to day practice – at the tables	Work on tables of 5–6 discussing each one's perspective on all principles in sequence	Copies of the key principles on the tables – enough copies
3.00	Ask for feedback from each of 4 tables. One spokesperson each – 5 minutes each Feedback noted on flip charts	Feedback	
3.15	Use audience response system to assess recall of key principles	Anonymous responses to questions	
3.30	Coffee break		
3.45	Recap on principles Again on tables asked to consider impact.	Listen Discuss	
4.10	Different spokesperson on each table.	Give feedback	
4.30	Audience response system	Anonymous answers	
4.45	Summarise key issues raised	Listen	
4.50	Recap on the session Ask each to state one thing they have learnt	Offer answer	
	Ask each to state on thing they still have questions/ unsure about	Offer answer	
5.00	Finish		

Lesson Plans

All of the above elements need to be incorporated into the lesson plan. It is useful particularly if embarking on a new session or course to write out the lesson plan with all the elements described above. In reality when facilitating or leading the course you may digress from the lesson plan and 'teach on the hoof'.

So the lesson plan is essentially a description of the activities within the lesson. The activities have to directly relate and map to the learning outcomes. Instructional design theory describes how to organise instruction to achieve the designated outcomes. There are four key aspects of instruction that any instructional designer needs to take into account (Okey 1991): clear and stated outcomes, the events to take place, the sequencing of these events, and appropriate activities.

Feedback

As mentioned above it is essential to obtain and give constructive feedback. We must be clear about the aims of our feedback questions. Are we seeking information about ourselves as educators or about the information we provide and whether it meets the learner's educational needs? Of course these two aspects are inter-related. For example, given similar content a learner will take away different messages from different educators. Nevertheless thinking about the distinction between feedback for the learner or educator will allow development of different feedback questions.

More traditional approaches to the obtaining of feedback have been based on questionnaires, which have included a combination of structured questions, open-ended responses and satisfaction scales. These approaches provide significant detail but are less helpful to the busy clinician-teacher. In addition, these techniques have been over-utilised resulting in the risk of 'feedback fatigue'. Learners need to understand and have confidence that their feedback will 'make a difference'.

Examples of feedback 'tools'

Feedback tools vary from low tech 'post it' notes through to Google forms. A few are described below.

Post it Notes

Post it notes or sticky notes are a simple, cheap and flexible way to obtain feedback. They are particularly useful if you want to gather a diverse range of opinions as in a listening exercise. They can be used at any point in session, for example, at the beginning to clarify learners expectations of the session.

One technique is to split learners into pairs and ask them to discuss a particular issue and jointly record their feedback on a maximum of two notes and stick up on a 'feedback wall'. The 'wall' can be a white board or a flip chart.

This allows for interaction, discussion and limiting the pairs to only two comments forces prioritisation of feedback.

The 'Stop, Start, Continue' technique is where every leaner is given two or three post it notes each and is asked to write down one thing the teacher should stop doing, one thing they should start doing, and one thing they should continue doing within the lesson. Feedback obtained by use of post it notes is usually concise and focused, which allows quick analysis by the teacher.

The One Minute Paper

The One Minute paper was first described by Wilson (1986) when at the beginning of a lecture he wrote two questions up on a board:

> *1) What is the most significant thing you learned today?*
> *2) What question is uppermost in your mind at the end of the class session? (Wilson 1986, p. 199)*

At the end of the lecture he gave students one minute to answer both questions.

The one minute paper has been used in a variety of learning environments and Whittard (2015) argues that the value of the use of this feedback technique is that it demonstrates respect for learners, creates an atmosphere of trust and encourages an active approach to learning.

Online Forms

Google, as an example, provides a range of online survey tools that can be easily adapted to meet whatever requirements you have for feedback. There are standard formats that can be used and the online versions allow the forms to be e-mailed to all learners and returned anonymously and the responses can be automatically collated and tabulated making analysis easy.

Audience Response Systems

There are a number of software packages available that allow the audiences in large or small groups to answer a number of questions throughout the session. Most systems allow anonymous polling with the ability to display polling results immediately. Tracking of individual responses is also possible with the 'clickers' registered to individuals. These can aid general discussion and hence interaction and can be used to gather feedback in regard to the learning process.

With each of these feedback techniques it is important that the correct questions are asked regarding content or teaching techniques so that the feedback loop can be closed. It is always useful to pilot the use of feedback questions and seek peer evaluation so that one's feedback is as useful as possible.

A Design Model for IPE

Reeves et al. (2007) described seven key factors in the planning and implementing of IPE in health care settings. These are high level factors that are a good starting point for any educationalists/trainers embarking on a new IPE course or reviewing and perhaps revising an established course. The authors use a widely accepted definition of IPE that has been subsequently ratified by the Centre for the Advancement of Interprofessional Education (CAIPE 2006).

The seven key factors described by Reeves et al. (2007) that need to be considered in designing and delivering any IPE learning experience are:

1 Promoting inter-professional interaction
2 Group dynamics: professional balance and stability
3 Relevance and status: ensuring IPE is valued
4 Expert facilitation
5 Facilitator support and training
6 Organisational implementation
7 Organisational support

Each of this will be explored in depth from an educational and a practical point of view.

Promoting Inter-professional Interaction

In order to learn from and about each other, interactive learning methods are essential. A range of interactive approaches are available.

Techniques to facilitate interaction:

Small group work
Problem- or case-based learning
Brainstorming
Buzz groups
Think, pair and share
Incident analysis
Quizzes
Question and answer

Small Group Work

Small group work and problem- or case-based learning in particular are effective teaching methods to facilitate interaction. Problem- and case-based learning are useful teaching methods within the IPE context. The next section will explore problem-based learning (PBL) as an example but a useful reference for case-based learning, equally appropriate for IPE is Williams (1992).

What is Problem-Based Learning?

PBL is a learner-centred approach to learning developed in McMaster University (Barrows and Tamblyn 1976). It is best to view PBL as a range of approaches underpinned by the essential elements of:

Patient problems as the starting point;

Learners work in small groups;

Analysis of the problem;

Identifying basic principles and concepts; and

Interactive learning.

Advantages of PBL

PBL in general is underpinned by a constructivist approach, which states that knowledge is constructed in the mind of the learner through perception of experiences (Schwandt 1994). Constructivism views that knowledge is not discovered but socially constructed. Dewey (1929) proposed that learners construct personal conceptual schemata (frameworks) in order to organise and retrieve information. Learning happens by activating appropriate schemata and incorporating new learning within the framework.

PBL is also learner-centred, encouraging learners have to take responsibility for their own learning, moving from passive receipt of information to active learning. The latter is a general term embedded in a number of learning methodologies. Denicolo et al. (1992) offered four distinct features of active learning:

1 A search for meaning and understanding;
2 Greater learner responsibility for learning;
3 Focus on knowledge and skills; and
4 An approach to learning that looks beyond the curriculum to lifelong learning.

Schmidt et al. (2011) suggest that PBL works as it encourages the activation of prior knowledge. This activation is facilitated by small group work that encourages opportunities for exploration and elaboration of the knowledge, thus leading to a deeper understanding. Also relevant problems enhance situational interest that enhances learning.

In designing an IPE course using PBL the following need to be considered:

1 Learning outcomes (dealt with earlier);
2 Designing the PBL 'Problems';
3 Facilitators/tutors;
4 Small groups;
5 Resources; and
6 Organisational issues.

Designing the PBL Problems

A practical approach to designing PBL problems describes seven qualities required of a PBL problem (Albanese and Mitchell 1993) and it is useful to use these as a framework to describe one's approach to the design of any course.

1 The first is to ensure that the problem is a common one that the learners would be expected to deal with in real clinical practice. This is essentially ensuring that the problem has relevance. One approach is to ensure that each of the problem scenarios is devised by an expert panel and is based on real patients. So the problems are both relevant to the 'curriculum' but are explicitly relevant to what the learners will be expected to face in the real world, in the clinical setting.

2 The problems should also be serious, have serious consequences depending on the management plan devised. That is, the outcome matters. For example, one of the problem scenarios may involve the learners exploring issues related to dignified death. So choosing serious and relevant problems that all learner professions will engage in equally is essential.

3 The problem scenarios should have a built in element of learning and understanding of primary prevention. With the scenarios, a common theme should be that early screening and clinicians having a high index of suspicion enable early diagnosis and a better outcome.

4 The problem should allow interdisciplinary and interprofessional aspects to be explored and have a broad base. With each problem there may be aspects of the need for services from the primary care team, pain clinics, surgical teams, third sector and patient-support groups.

5 The problems will map directly to the learning outcomes as above.

6 The problems should present a concrete task or tasks for the learners to work and focus on. This is a key element and the problems should be designed so that specific tasks and subtasks are required.

7 The problems should also have a level of complexity that is appropriate for the learners' prior experience and knowledge. It is essential that if one is targeting a group of experienced clinicians to ensure that the problems will reflect the complexities of the learners' clinical interactions on the 'coal face'.

Facilitators

Not all teachers or trainers are comfortable with the demands of a PBL approach. In an ideal world, all health educators would have a wide range of characteristics but the reality is that being an effective teacher/trainer is a process of continuous improvement (Ralhan et al. 2012).

There is a tendency for medical teachers as an example, to teach as they were taught (Irby 1996). The role of the facilitator is intrinsically different to that of the traditional lecturer. There is a unique set of competencies associated with a PBL facilitator. In addition to the having skills in small group facilitation, and an understanding of the wider programme and the specific learning outcomes there is debate in regard to their position or otherwise as the content experts.

There are two positions. In the original McMaster curriculum where PBL originated (Wood 2003) there was a conscious decision that the facilitators did not, and should not be content experts. This was to reduce the temptation of the experts 'lecturing' the learners (the traditional knowledge transmission interaction). Others argue that the best outcomes are achieved if subject experts are trained in facilitation techniques (Davis et al. 1992). Although the learner group may be made up of experienced clinicians they may still have had limited exposure to PBL. They will require further support including a study guide to help them manage their own learning in an effective manner (Laidlaw and Harden 1990).

Small groups for PBL

There a number of key questions to ask when organising and managing small groups including the size, composition, assignment of roles and time management. This is of particular importance in IPE. The optimum number in a small group is considered to be seven with evidence that if the number is above ten this leads to poorer quality interaction (Hughes and Lucas 1997). Depending on the type of course or programme, in other words, the mix of potential learner groups, the logistics may mean that one cannot allocate the natural 'teams' into one PBL group so a mix across may be required.

Considering the multiprofessional nature of the entire cohort, it can be important to assign individuals to groups to ensure a balance. One can always alter this based on observations of the group dynamics. It is important to ensure engagement of all members and if some dominate or monopolise then re-assignment may help.

Each of the problem scenarios should have explicit role assignments and if the learners are relatively inexperienced with PBL one can assign specific administrative roles of recorder and action list generator (Barrows 1985). In planning PBL it is best if role assignments are planned so that all learners take part and 'play' each other's roles thus enhancing each groups' understanding of each other.

It is also useful to provide a set of ground rules for the use of technology, time management and breaks.

Resources

Physical resources requirements will need to be built into the plan for delivery of any PBL course. One needs to be specific in regard to this and plan ahead. Moving from a traditional lecture-based programme there may have been a requirement for a 50-seater lecture theatre and one lecturer for a morning session. If the cohort remains at 50 but using a PBL approach there will be a need for 7 group rooms if one adheres to 7 in each group. Compromise may be required on the course organiser's part if the ideal physical facilities are not available. Managing the learning environment 'on the hoof' is an important skill in any teaching methodology but particularly with small-group PBL.

Organisational issues
Moving even just one course from a traditional lecture-based delivery model to PBL will have major resource requirements for one's organisation. The manpower may have been identified previously, using more traditional methods. This may have been assessed as, say, two tutors and a part time administrator. Moving to PBL may then require seven facilitators who are trained, generation of lesson plans, study guides for the learners, and more logistical challenges such as access to kettles, coffee and so on.

Summary of PBL approaches
The principles that one should use to re-design a course in order to facilitate using a PBL approach have been described in the preceding subsections. The key elements are starting with relevant and important 'problems' that map to the learning outcomes. The education strategies include small group work with trained content expert facilitators. A PBL approach facilitates a learner-centred and interactive learning experience.

Brainstorming
In small or even larger group sessions, brainstorming is a useful tool to facilitate creative problem solving, enhance social cohesion and increase the overall creativity of the group. Osborn (1963) is frequently attributed with originating this technique. In practice a question is posed to all the members of the group. The participants discuss the question/issue posed and in a free flowing way offering ideas. Brainstorming works best if some principles are adhered to;
Go for quantity … the more ideas the more chance of finding the best solution
No criticism … no judgements should be made on any ideas offered
Encourage wild ideas … these may stimulate further new ideas
Combine and improve ideas

Buzz Groups
A buzz group is a small group, usually of three to six participants who are given an assignment to complete in a short time period. Each buzz group records their output and then reports to the larger group when the task is finished. They are a useful tool to use to help ownership of learning to move

from the tutor/trainer to the learners themselves. According to Thelen (1967), this technique is also useful for:
Getting the learners started on a new problem;
Overcome a feeling of apathy or inertia or to refocus the learners; and
To test out new ideas

Think, Pair and Share

With this teaching strategy the tutor trainers acts as a facilitator and poses a question to the group. Each learner is given some time to think through the question and is then paired off with a peer and they share their thinking. This allows social interaction, sharing of ideas in a safe space and both communication and listening skills.

The next step could be each pair sharing key agreed points with the wider group or then pairs joining and repeating the process. This is an extremely simple technique that be used at any point in a session and is particularly helpful for the tutor/trainer to have a better understanding of the learners' thinking and views.

Incident Analysis

This is a widely used technique as a way of allowing learners to reflect and make sense of events. It is a widely used lifelong learning tool (Henderson et al. 2002). As a result of reflection, gaps in knowledge or understanding can be identified. One method is to ask each learner to think about an incident beforehand and be prepared to share it with the group. Each learner then in turn describes what happened and as a facilitator, one asks them to identify their initial thoughts and feelings. The stage after that is to facilitate the learner to reflect and evaluate the event … the 'why do you think it happened' question, and then the conclusion … 'what did you learn or importantly what gaps do you perceive?' … hence generating areas for development.

Group Dynamics: Professional Balance and Stability

There are a number of steps that one needs to take in determining the composition of groups when using an IPE type approach. The starting point is the aims and specific learning outcomes as discussed earlier. It is important to have a clear understanding of what IPE type learning has been undertaken/ experienced by the groups you have in mind. There is a real need to consider very carefully the professional and discipline balance within the learners' cohort and then in specific small groups if that is your teaching methodology. As a result of the traditional hierarchical relationships that may have existed between the professions over many years (Hammick et al. 2007) it is essential that no single profession is or is seen to be dominant in any group work, scenarios and pre- or debriefing. This is not just about the numbers of each profession but also addressing issues such as ensuring the scheduling of learning is equitable.

These issues are echoed from published studies looking at the barriers and facilitators of interprofessional team work in health care settings. Xyrichis and Lowton (2008) identified the following factors as important:
Team premises;
Team size and Team composition;
Organisation supporting team meetings;
Clear goals and objectives; and
Audit of activity.

In order to design an IPE course it is essential to understand the intended audience, consultants, staff and associate specialist grade, higher trainees, nurse specialists, physiotherapists and non- clinical staff and refocus your strategy for advertising. One option is to target natural teams in specific health environments and allocate them to small groups based on their department. The disadvantage of this is that the established dynamics in these 'natural' teams may act as a barrier to genuine interaction.

Relevance and Status: Ensuring IPE is Valued

If learning is highly valued then there is more likelihood of learners perceiving or feeling that it is of significance to them personally. The concept of significant learning is characterised by:

> *some kind of lasting change that is important in terms of the learner's life.*
> (Fink 2003, p. 295)

Participants in IPE have reported gaining most from the experience when there is genuine engagement with other learners from other professions working jointly on a relevant problem (Gilligan et al. 2014). Hence, participants' involvement will be enhanced if IPE is perceived as relevant. When using a PBL approach, it is key that the problem scenarios are pitched at the correct level of complexity mapped to real and 'hot' issues in the clinical environment.

It is important to ensure that the facilitators are trained in IPE as described but more importantly that they are also seen as experts with authority. Also it is always useful to ensure that continuing professional development points will be gained.

Another tactic will be to market the course and re-brand emphasising the IPE nature and enlisting the support of Royal Colleges and other professional bodies involved.

It is important to recognise the importance of informal IPE. This is the informal social interaction built into any learning experience, coffee breaks and so on. These opportunities to interact can be extremely positive and hence have a real positive impact on the formal IPE. Studies have shown that these social factors played an important role within the wider experience of learners (Reeves 2000).

Expert Facilitation

The skill set, attitude, competencies and confidence required for IPE facilitators is different to those in other settings (Holland 2002). The demands of IPE groups can be high and experience in dealing with possible dynamics that manifest are key.

The facilitators must be aware of the interprofessional conflicts both more generally and between individuals. Ideally, these conflicts should be used to develop and maintain a team ethos (Headrick et al. 1998).

It is clear that the skills and competencies are different and not all experts, in this case experts in assessment in the work place, per se will be able to facilitate effectively. If using a PBL or case-based approach there is an argument that the best outcomes are achieved if subject experts are trained in facilitation techniques (Davis et al. 1992). This is a key issue and flows into one of Reeves and colleagues' other factors of facilitator support. These development programmes are crucial to prepare tutors particularly those inexperienced in IPL settings.

Facilitator Support and Training

Irrespective of the teaching methodology, it is essential that tutors and facilitators are supported and provided with on-going professional development opportunities. Given the specific and significantly different demands of facilitating in small groups, using a PBL or case-based approach within an IPE model it is imperative that facilitators are selected and supported (Freeth et al. 2005).

Facilitation differs from leading or directing teaching. The University of Toronto, Centre for Education (2018) defines facilitation as:

> the process of helping groups or individuals to learn, find solutions or reach consensus without imposing or dictating an outcome. Facilitation works to empower individuals or groups to learn for themselves or find their own answers.

It is well recognised (Anderson et al. 2013) that faculty development is essential for ensuring effective high quality IPE and that there is a particular mind set: that is for faculty to think outside of their own professional silo and the inherent boundaries these set. The aim is for the IPE facilitator to act as a co-creator of IP knowledge.

Nicol and Forman (2014) suggested that IPE was most effective if facilitators tailored the experience to meet the needs of specific clinical placement and the specific learning needs of learners. So, according to Chipchase et al. 2012, the attributes required of an IPE facilitator include:

Inspiration;

Reassurance;

An understanding of team formation;

An understanding of group dynamics; and

The ability to resolve conflict.

Therefore on-going support and development for IPE facilitators is essential and will require planning and resources.

Organisational Implementation

All educational organisations, at whatever level the learning is pitched, need to plan IPE in a co-ordinated manner. One key question for any organisation is the timing of the IPE with a course or programme. There is evidence that some students at undergraduate level have preconceived professional stereotypes that can act as barriers to IPE. The argument there is that IPE should be embedded in programmes as early as possible. On the other hand others have argued that IPE is best positioned post qualification so that participants have a clear idea of their uni-professional roles and identity and hence are best placed to understand how their role fits in the wider health and social care system and hence how other professions fit.

Organisational Support

Planning and implementing effective IPE is clearly complex and will, therefore, require support from the home organisation, university, heath boards, trusts or others.

There can arise a number of organisational barriers to the delivery of IPE. Undergraduate (UG) can be more problematic as a result of more institutional barriers such as timetabling a number of UG programmes on multiple sites. In general the barriers within organisations can be:

Imbalance in learner numbers … too many of one profession;

Learning space pressure … small group PBL needs rooms; and

Access to IT and study space may be issues.

Extra institutional barriers (Pirrie et al. 1998) can include out-of-sync revalidation cycles, for example nursing in the UK is three years and for doctors the cycle is every five years. Separate and competing funding streams can also lead to barriers in supporting IPE activity across professions and or organisations. Disparate professional bodies with perceptions of conflicting agendas can also lead to lack of meaningful engagement.

In summary, the paper published by Reeves et al. (2007) provides a useful framework indicating high-level factors that need to be considered in designing and delivering effective IPE, where the key concept is to learn from and about each other. One risk in ill-designed IPE learning experiences is that the different professionals present focus solely on acquiring the same knowledge or skills. The real difference with IPE is that they learn from each other and learn about each other's roles, skills and attitudes.

The Use of Distance Learning in IPE

The use of online resources to support and enhance the learning experience has grown in recent years. Distance learning (DL) also referred to as distance education and distributed learning involves five qualities that help distinguish it from other forms of instruction (Keegan 1996):
1 the quasi-permanent separation of the teachers/trainers and learners;
2 the influence of an education organisation on the planning, preparation and provision of support for learners;
3 the use of technical media;
4 the provision of two-way communication; and
5 the quasi-permanent absence of learning groups.
So, DL can be viewed as a teaching methodology to deliver learning to an individual or group of learners. These learners do not necessarily need to be physically present in a traditional classroom, or seminar room. The approach can be synchronous, with communications in real time, such as chat rooms. With asynchronous methods communications are out of sync in time and place, with emails being the obvious example.

An example of the use of a virtual community (VC) combined with a narrative or story telling approach is the Stilwel project (Giddens and Walsh 2010). This is a multimedia VC that tells the story of residents in three different roads in the Stilwel area of Brigstow. Stilwel was designed as an IP learning environment where students can be exposed to challenging scenarios, for example child protection issues. The approach is based in reality and explicit and difficult narratives are worked through.

If one uses online techniques within a DL approach to support the small group work there are however specific issues to consider.

Some benefits of online collaboration
1 Convenience;
2 Engagement;
3 Ownership; and
4 Audit trails.

Convenience

Using online teaching methods affords significant flexibility and convenience for both facilitators and learners. Participation can be programmed to suit the needs of busy clinicians and negates the need for all learners to 'attend' a physical venue. Contributions to the group's work can be done from home, or any other remote location including across the world. So learning and instruction can be undertaken at a time and place that suits the individual.

Most multifunction platforms allow the use of a range of different functions such as email, document sharing, surveying and meetings on one website, rather than using separate tools for each task. If there is a need to share documents, this can be done in a single place online and sharing access to useful resources can be more effective than using email. Automated notifications can be set up to keep all group members informed of events so that you don't need to login regularly.

Engagement

Engagement of, and interaction between learners is key to the success of any learning experience and particularly so for IPE activity. Used effectively, the currently available online collaborative tools can facilitate active engagement from all learners. Each learner can be allocated specific tasks to be undertaken on behalf of the group and each participant's roles can be made explicit to all learners. The online environment does encourage quieter members of the group to share their views and engage with the experience more than they might have done in face-to-face 'classroom' scenarios.

Ownership of Learning

Ownership of learning is key to motiving learners. The use of online tools can facilitate enhanced group and individual ownership. Roles and responsibilities in learning groups can be discussed and agreed and decisions on these taken jointly via Wiki or chat-room type functions. As the effectiveness of any learning but particularly IPE is enhanced by clear ownership this is extremely useful.

The social interaction afforded by online learning can also help the learning experience. This is particularly relevant if the learners are based in distributed sites over a wide area. Online learning will enable interaction on a more frequent basis than would be possible if having to rely on face-to-face meetings.

Audit Trails

It is important for both the learners and the facilitators/teachers to have ready access to an archive of papers, summary of discussions and chat room trails to rely on. Most collaborative tools will provide these functions and they are particularly useful for any learners who are unable to participate in certain meetings for a period of time – whilst on annual leave for example.

Challenges of Online Learning

Online learning is a tool to enhance learning but one must be aware of some challenges, which include:

1 Using technology because it is there;
2 Access and support; and
3 Technological Redundancy.

Using Technology Because It is There

The first step if one is considering using technology is to return to the aims and learning objectives and consider in what ways technology could help deliver those objectives for the learners. If one has access to online resources it is very easy to lose sight of the purpose in collaborating online. The risk is that technology starts to determine the learning.

It is vital to map the learning objectives to the online teaching methods available to you. It is important to remember that collaborative working online requires a set of rules similar to those needed if you are using face-to-face meetings. There is a need to address team dynamics, rules of communication, roles and responsibilities and time management.

Access and Support

With any new online tool there is a need for investment of time in getting to know it's functions and feel familiar with it. The learners may have had experience of the tools before or they may be completely new to the whole field of online learning. These differences will need to be taken into account. Access to the correct specification of software needed to run programmes may vary and depending on the learners' location, access and speed of broadband will vary.

There is also a need for ongoing technical advice in case there are malfunctions. Some software products have easily accessible online manuals or even telephone support services, not all do. You will need to take these issues into consideration when choosing which program to use.

Technological Redundancy

New online technologies evolve very quickly. There is always a temptation to upgrade to the latest version of a programme that has been used before. There are inherent risks in this as companies are constantly upgrading and the upgrade may not meet your learners' needs in the same way that the older version does quite successfully. Having a good working relationship with your institute's IT department is vital.

Lessons from IPE Using Simulation

Boet et al. (2014) described 12 tips for simulation IPE but even though their focus was on simulation education, the principles are transferable across any teaching methodology and will be discussed briefly.

1 Focus on the 'interprofessional'.
2 Anticipate complex logistical challenges.
3 Find your interprofessional simulation champions.
4 Balance diversity with equity.
5 Develop scenarios that are relevant to all professions.
6 Be mindful of sociological fidelity.
7 Put all the professions on the same page: the importance of pre-briefing.
8 Beware of interprofessional debriefing challenges.
9 Use simulation to add value within the broader interprofessional curriculum.
10 Focus the assessment on the team.
11 Support the interprofessional simulation educators.
12 Interprofessional simulated learning is under researched: use teaching opportunities to foster research.

These are broadly in line with Reeves et al. (2007) with the added focus on simulation.

Chapter Summary

It is important to have a framework or plan in designing and delivering any learning experience. Considering the added complexities of IPE these are increasingly important.

In this chapter basic concepts are explored set against the IPE background including learning needs analysis, aims, learning objectives, lesson plans and feedback techniques. A detailed sample lesson plan is described.

In regard to the design and implementation of IPE seven key principles are explored in detail (Reeves et al. 2007).

The importance of designing the learning so as to maximise the opportunity for IP interaction is stressed and techniques that can be used to facilitate this including small group work. The principles underpinning PBL are explored as just one example of using small groups as to facilitate enhanced interaction thus increasing engagement of learners and affording them more ownership of their learning.

References

Albanese, M.A. and Mitchell, S. (1993). Problem-based learning: a review of literature on its outcomes and implementation issues. *Academic Medicine* 68: 53–81.

Anderson, L., Hean, S., O'Halloran, C. et al. (2013). Faculty development for interprofessional education and practice. In: *Faculty Development in the Health Professions* (ed. Y. Steinert), 287–310. Dordrecht: Springer.

Barrows, H.S. (1985). *How to Design a Problem-Based Curriculum for the Preclinical Years*. New York: Springer.

Barrows, H.S. and Tamblyn, R.M. (1976). An evaluation of problem-based learning in small groups utilising a simulated patient. *Journal of Medical Education* 51: 52–54.

Boet, S., Bould, D.M., Burn, C.L. et al. (2014). Twelve tips for a successful interprofessional team-based high-fidelity simulation education session. *Medical Teacher* 36 (10): 853–857.

Boyd, E. and Fales, A. (1983). Reflective learning: key to learning from experience. *Journal of Humanistic Psychology* 23: 99–117.

CAIPE (2006). CAIPE re-issues its statement on the definition and principles of interprofessional education. *CAIPE Bulletin* 26: 3.

Chipchase, J., Allen, S., Eley, D. et al. (2012). Interprofessional supervision in an intercultural context: A qualitative study. *Journal of Interprofessional Care* 26 (6): 465–471.

Davis, W.K., Naim, R., Paine, M.E. et al. (1992). Effects of expert and non-expert facilitators on the small group process and on student performance. *Academic Medicine* 67: 407–474.

Denicolo, P., Entwistle, N., and Hounsell, D. (1992). What is active learning? In: *Effective Learning and Teaching in Higher Education Module 1, 54*. Sheffield: CVCP Universities' Staff Development and Training Unit.

Dewey, J. (1929). *The Quest for Certainty*. New York: Minton.

Fink, L.D. (2003). *Creating Significant Learning Experience: An Integrated Approach to Designing College Courses*. San Francisco, CA: Jossey-Bass Publishers.

Freeth, D., Hammock, M., Reeves, S. et al. (2005). *Effective Interprofessional Education: Development, Delivery and Evaluation*. London, UK: Blackwell Science.

Giddens, J. and Walsh, M. (2010). Collaborating across the pond; the diffusion of virtual communities for nursing education. *Journal of Nursing Education* 49 (8): 449–455.

Gilligan, C., Outram, S., and Levett-Jones, T. (2014). Recommendations from recent graduates in medicine, nursing and pharmacy on improving interprofessional education in university programs: A qualitative study. *BMC Medical Education* 14: 52.

Hammick, M., Freeth, D., Koppel, I. et al. (2007). A best evidence systematic review of interprofessional education: BEME Guide no.9. *Medical Teacher* 29 (8): 735–751.

Harden, R. (2000). The integration ladder: a tool for curriculum planning and evaluation. *Medical Education* 34: 551–557.

Headrick, L., Wilcock, P., and Batalden, P. (1998). Interprofessional working and continuing medical education. *British Medical Journal* 316: 771–774.

Henderson, J., Dickson, P., Hess, M. et al. (2002). Global production networks and the analysis of economic development. *Review of International Political Economy* 9 (3): 436–464.

Holland, K. (2002). Interprofessional education and practice: the role of the teacher/facilitator. *Nurse Education Practice* 2: 221–222.

Hughes, L. and Lucas, J. (1997). An evaluation of problem based learning in the multi professional education curriculum for the health professions. *Journal of Interprofessional Care* 11: 77–88.

Irby, D.M. (1996). Models of faculty development for problem-based learning. *Advances in Health Sciences Education* 1: 69–81.

Keegan, D. (1996). *Foundations of Distance Education*, 3e. London: Routledge.

Knowles, M., Swanson, R., and Holton, E. (2011). *The Adult Learner: The Definitive Classic in Adult Education and Human Resource Development*, 7e. Amsterdam: Elsevier:.

Knowles, M.S. (1980). *The Modern Practice of Adult Education: From Pedagogy to Andragogy*, 2e. New York: Cambridge Books.

Kolb, D.A. (1984). *Experiential Learning Experience as a Source of Learning and Development*. New Jersey: Prentice Hall.

Krathwohl, D.R. (2002). A revision of Bloom's taxonomy: an overview. *Theory Into Practice* 41 (4): 212–218.

Laidlaw, J.M. and Harden, R.M. (1990). What is … a study guide. *Medical Teacher* 12: 94–101.

Laxdal, O. (1982). Needs assessment in continuing medical education: a practical guide. *Journal of Medical Education* 57: 827–834.

Lockyer, J. (1998). Needs assessment: lesson learned. *Journal of Continuing Education in the Health Professions* 18: 190–192.

Luft, J. and Ingham, H. (1950). *The Johari window, a graphic model of interpersonal awareness*. In: *Proceedings of the western training laboratory in group development*. Los Angeles: UCLA.

Moon, J. (1999). *Learning Journals: A Handbook for Academics, Students and Professional Development*. London: Kogan Page.

Nicol, P.W. and Forman, D. (2014). Attributes of effective interprofessional placement facilitation. *Journal of Research in Interprofessional Practice and Education* 4 (20): 1–11.

Okey, J.R. (1991). Procedures of lesson design Ch. 6. In: *Instructional Design: Principles and Applications*, 2e (ed. L.J. Briggs, K.L. Gustafson and M.H. Tillman), 192–208. Englewood Cliffs, NJ: Education Technology Publications.

Osborn, A.F. (1963). *Applied Imagination: Principles and Procedures of Creative Problem Solving*, Third Revisede. New York, NY: Charles Scribner's Sons.

Pirrie, A., Wilson, V., Harden, R.M. et al. (1998). AMEE Guide No. 12: multiprofessional education part 2 – promoting cohesive practice in health care. *Medical Teacher* 20: 409–416.

Ralhan, S., Bhogal, P., Bhatnagar, G., et al. (2012). Effective teaching skills – how to be a better medical educator. *BMJ Careers* 344, https://doi.org/10.1136/bmj.e765 (accessed 18 September 2018).

Reeves, S. (2000). Commnuity-based interprofessional education for medical, nursing and dental students. *Health Social Care Community* 4: 269–276.

Reeves, S., Goldman, J., Gilbert, J. et al. (2011). A scoping review to improve conceptual clarity of interprofessional interventions. *Journal of Interprofessional Care* 25: 167–174.

Reeves, S., Goldman, J., and Oandasan, I. (2007). Key factors in planning and implementing interprofessional education in health care settings. *Journal of Allied Health* 36 (4): 231–235.

Sargeant, J., Armson, H., Chesluk, B. et al. (2010). The processes and dimensions of informed self-assessment: a conceptual model. *Academic Medicine* 85 (7): 1212–1220.

Schmidt, H.G., Rotgans, J.I., and Yew, E.H.J. (2011). The process of problem-based leanring: what works and why. *Medical Education* 45: 792–806.

Schön, D.A. (1983). *The Reflective Practitioner: How Professionals Think in Action.* New York: Basic Books.

Schwandt, T.A. (1994). Constructivist, interpretivist approaches to human enquiry. In: *Handbook of Qualitative Research* (ed. D.K. Denzin and T.S. Lincoln), 118–137. Thousand Oaks, CA: Sage.

Thelen, H.A. (1967). *Dynamics of Groups at Work.* Chicago, IL: Chicago University of Chicago Press.

University of Toronto, Centre for Interprofessional Education. http://www.ipe. utoronto.ca/curriculum/facilitators/facilitators (accessed: 30 June 2018).

Waller, K.V. (1962). Writing instructional objectives. National Accrediting Agency for Clinical Laboratory Sciences. https://www.sc.edu/about/offices_and_divisions/cte/ teaching_resources/docs/writing_instructional_objectives.pdf (accessed: 30 June 2018).

Whittard, D. (2015). Reflections on the one minute paper. *International Review of Economics Education* 20: 1–12.

Williams, S.M. (1992). Putting case-based instruction into context: examples from legal and medical education. *Journal of the Learning Sciences* 2: 367–427.

Wilson, R.C. (1986). Improving faculty teaching: effective use of student evaluations and consultants. *The Journal of Higher Education* 57 (2): 196–211.

Wood, D.F. (2003). ABC of learning and teaching in medicine: problem based learning. *British Medical Journal* 326: 328–330.

Xyrichis, A. and Lowton, K. (2008). What fosters or prevents interprofessional teamworking in primary and community care? A literature review. *International Journal of Nursing Studies* 45: 140–153.

Xyrichis, A., Reeves, S., and Zwarenstein, M. (2017). Examining the nature of interprofessional practice: an initial framework validation and creation of the Interprofessional Activity Classification Tool (InterPACT). *Journal of Interprofessional Care* https://doi. org/10.1080/13561820.2017.1408576.

Chapter 5 **Examples of Interprofessional Education in Practice**

Introduction

There are a range of one off initiatives and pilots and evaluation in the field of Interprofessional Education (IPE). In addition, there are organisations, real physical and virtual entities that have set the conditions for the enhancement of IPE through specific initiatives that have grown and led to institutional, regional and global change for the benefit of patients. This chapter is in three main sections:

Organisations across the world that support IPE;

Journals and other publications supporting IPE; and

Examples of organisations with major IPE transformation programmes and those within or facilitating a community of practice in IPE.

Organisations that Support IPE

Australasian Interprofessional Practice and Education Network (AIPPEN)

In the early 2000s, there was recognition in Australia and New Zealand of the need to promote IP Learning (IPL) at a local, institutional and governmental level but that there were insufficient structures in place to facilitate this.

There was the Rural Interprofessional Practice and Education Network (RIPEN) that was established in 2004 but no overarching organisation. In addition, there was a real sense that any IPE initiatives were driven from the bottom up by educationalists and clinicians on the ground rather than from central government policy. Set against this background proposals were published (Nisbet et al. 2007) to set up the Australasian Interprofessional Practice and Education Network (AIPPEN), which exists to provide a virtual meeting place for clinicians, researchers, scholars, patients, carers and managers to

How to Succeed at Interprofessional Education, First Edition. Peter Donnelly.
© 2019 John Wiley & Sons Ltd. Published 2019 by John Wiley & Sons Ltd.

interact and promote IPE and collaborative practice. The focus is improving patient outcomes across the health and social care sectors.

From its web site (https://www.anzahpe.org/aippen, accessed: 30 June 2018) AIPPEN aims to:

> promote the development of a network that can link health professional education and care sectors, universities, vocational education and training sector, government, practitioners and service users (patients);
> organize a series of seminars and conferences to share information and experiences;
> influence workforce policy and practice change in Australia and New Zealand;
> encourage research, evaluation and collaboration between different teams that can demonstrate the health-care and economic advantages of interprofessional learning;
> disseminate information on interprofessional learning.

Canadian Interprofessional Health Collaborative (CIHC)

The educators in the Faculty of Medicine, McGill University, Montreal, Quebec, Canada have been working together since approximately 2008 developing an IP heath collaborative. This has developed into a pan-Canadian collaborative of partners promoting Interprofessional Education for Collaborative Patient-Centred Practice (IECPCP) with the goal of improving health education leading to improved health outcomes for individual patients and the wider population of Canada.

CIHC's focus is on acting as a hub to share best practices in interprofessional education and collaborative practice recognising that patient care is improved if health professionals work together. Membership of CIHC is open to all at no charge.

Taken from the website (https://www.cihc.ca/, accessed: 30 June 2018) CIHC aims to:

> facilitate knowledge production, exchange and application in interprofessional education and collaborative practice;
> foster strategic and innovative partnerships that enable interprofessional collaboration in education, research and practice;
> promote a coordinated approach to curriculum development and reform;
> articulate, advance, and advocate a research and evaluation agenda for interprofessional education and collaborative practice;
> develop support for leadership in interprofessional education and collaborative practice;
> build the Canadian Interprofessional Health Collaborative and model interprofessional collaborative approaches within and among organizations and sectors.

The European Interprofessional Education Network (EIPEN)

The European Interprofessional Education Network (EIPEN) was launched in 2004 following a research project to support IPE in the UK led by the Subject Centre for Health Sciences and Practice, Kings College, London. EIPEN has undergone a number of iterations. The challenges of working across different political, educational and linguistic boundaries has to some extent hampered progress that might have otherwise been made. Currently EIPEN is supported across Europe with higher education and employer partners from Belgium, Finland, Greece, Hungary, Ireland, Poland, Slovenia, Sweden and the United Kingdom.

On the EIPEN website (https://www.eipen.eu/, accessed: 30 June 2018) it states;

> *EIPEN has two interlinked aims to:*
> *develop a transnational network of universities and employers in the participating countries; and*
> *promote good practices in interprofessional learning and teaching in health-care.*

Nordic Interprofessional Network (NIPNet)

The Nordic Interprofessional Network (NIPNet) was launched in Norway in 2001. The initial aim was to get exponents of IPE together to share ideas and develop a mutual support network across health and social care.

NIPNet's focus is to act as a platform to promote education, practice and research primarily for Nordic educators, practitioners and researchers in the fields of health. The members represent interprofessional education initiatives in Denmark, Finland, Norway and Sweden. The organisation is run by a board with up to five representatives from each Nordic country.

NIPNet supports annual conferences that alternate between the Nordic countries. The business of NIPNet is to create partnerships between individuals and organisations across the borders of Nordic countries with the purpose of developing IPE and interprofessional collaboration (IPC) practices for the benefit of patients. There is no formal membership of NIPNet as such with a simple sign-in that results in you receiving newsletters and posts. NIPNet is a member of the World Coordinating Committee All Together Better Health (WCC-ATBH).

Centre for the Advancement of Interprofessional Education (CAIPE)

The Centre for the Advancement of Interprofessional Education (CAIPE) was originally an independent UK charity, legally founded in 1987. Its origins began several years prior to that with the piloting of IPE in the London borough of Enfield. The organisation has evolved and undergone a number of iterations expanding from its initial focus on primary care to include individuals from across the health and voluntary care sector in the UK with a growing international representation. It is now a membership body with some 300 fee paying members who form a network of mutual support and interest.

CAIPE is a national and international resource for IPE across the health and social care workplace and for universities providing education and training. In addition to promoting all aspects of IPE CAIPE's focus is as an enabler of change in this arena. From the web site (https://www.caipe.org/, accessed: 30 June 2018):

> *We are a community committed to collaborative working across health and social care and related services. CAIPE aims to promote and develop interprofessional education, research, learning and practice globally.*
>
> *We recognise interprofessional education as occasions when members or students of two or more professions learn with, from and about each other to improve collaboration and the quality of care and services.*
>
> *We are one of the leading organisations in the global development of interprofessional education and collaborative practice through learning together to work together.*
>
> *We support students, academics, practitioners, researchers and people who use services by sharing information and enabling networking opportunities.*

World Coordinating Committee All Together Better Health

The World Coordinating Committee All Together Better Health (WCC-ATBH) is a collaboration of worldwide organisations with the focus on promoting and developing IPE and IPP in health and social care. Through member networks and the ATBH conferences the IPE agenda is enhanced. The ATBH works with other human health organisations such as the World Health Organisation (WHO) and the United Nations Educational, Scientific and Cultural Organization (UNESCO). All of the above organisations are member networks.

In addition there are a number of education organisations that although having medical in the title are increasingly supportive of a Multiprofessional (MP) approach and those that support this agenda. These include the following.

The Association for the Study of Medical Education (ASME) was established in 1957 and aims to help meet the needs of teachers, trainers and learners across medical education by supporting research-informed best practice. Its membership focuses on all who are involved in medical education and training and it provides CPD, leadership development and research in medical education networks. Although UK based, it is internationally facing and publishes with Wiley two education journals, the monthly *Medical Education* and bi-monthly *Clinical Teacher*.

The Association for Medical Education in Europe (AMEE), founded in Copenhagen in 1972, aims to promote excellence in education in healthcare professions across a broad spectrum. AMEE is the regional association of the World Federation of Medical Education. It is a worldwide organisation with members across 90 countries.

The Academy of Medical Educators (AoME) was established in 2006 as a multiprofessional organisation with the aim of providing leadership and promoting standards in medical education. Its focus is on medicine, dentistry and veterinary professionals. It has developed the professional standards that formed the backbone of those adopted by the General Medical Council (GMC).

The Association for Simulated Practice in Healthcare (ASPiH) is dedicated to improving patient care and professional performance by the use of simulated practice and technology-enhanced learning. It is a not-for-profit membership association with a focus on multiprofessional and team working.

Publications Supporting IPE

In this section, a brief summary of key publications that directly focus on and support IPE will be given. Where appropriate the impact factor and five years impact factor is given.

The impact factor is a measure of the frequency that the 'average article' has been cited and the five years impact is this measure over a five-year period.

Journal of Interprofessional Care

The *Journal of Interprofessional Care* began as *Holistic Medicine* from 1986 taking on it's current title in 1992. The journal has an international reputation as a leading authority in publishing high quality papers with a sole focus on IPE and training. The journal publishes papers across the spectrum from policy pieces, research, evaluations and descriptive works. It welcomes submissions that help inform collaboration in education and practice across all professions including medicine, nursing, veterinary science, allied health, public health, social care and related professions.

The journal's scope has widened in recent years with contributions from a range of fields including child care, older people, criminal justice, education for special needs, palliative care, and learning disabilities.

The types of articles published are:
Peer reviewed original research articles
Systematic/analytical reviews
Theoretical papers
Peer reviewed short reports (research in progress or completed or innovations)
The impact factor is 2.205
The five-year impact factor is 2.456

Journal of Continuing Education in the Health Professions

This is a quarterly peer reviewed journal previously published by Wiley now by Wolters Kluwer. It is the official journal of the Alliance for Continuing Education in the Health Professions, the Association for Hospital Medical Education, and the Society for Academic Continuing Medical Education. It's focus is on studies/articles relevant to the theory, practice and policy development for continuing education and continuing professional education in the health sciences. The focus is medicine, nursing and other health care professionals. Issues contain the following types of articles: original research with a lesson for practice focus, innovations in continuing education, and book reviews. Although this journal does not explicitly focus on IPE it's remit is broad and often publishes studies in this field.

The types of articles published are:
Original research
Innovations in continuing education
Book reviews

Journal of Research in Interprofessional Practice and Education

The *Journal of Research in Interprofessional Practice and Education* is a peer-reviewed open-access journal that publishes a wide range articles supporting evidence-based knowledge to inform IP practice, education and research.

The main aims of the journal are (from web site, https://www.jripe.org/index.php/journal, accessed: 30 June 2018):

1 *To improve understanding of the processes involved in IPE and how they are linked to specific outcomes defined at the level of the patient, the family, the health care team, the health care organization, and the community level;*
2 *To stimulate the development of the evidence related to these processes;*
3 *To facilitate knowledge exchange between those who fund and conduct research, and those who use and apply research in practice and policy settings.*

Types of articles published are:
Theory
Methodology
Empirical research
Reflection and hypotheses
Book reviews

Focus on Health Professional Education:
A Multi-Professional Journal

Focus on Health Professional Education (FoHPE) is the official journal of the Australian and New Zealand Association for Health Professional Educators (ANZAHPE). It is a peer-refereed journal that was formally established in 1998, and is published by the Association to promote, support and advance education in all the health professions.

The journal's focus is on multiprofessional education in health. Although the main focus is around the region of the Western Pacific areas of Australia and New Zealand and South East Asia it maintains an international approach.

Types of article published are:
Original Research
Scholarly Papers
Systematic reviews
Reports on educational innovations
Short discussion papers on issues of current interest
In addition, the journal will consider Innovative Teaching and Learning Projects (ITLP), giving authors the opportunity to disseminate their innovations in a brief report without producing a full research paper. This format includes small-scale innovations in healthcare education and is particularly designed for emerging 'hot topics'.

Health and Interprofessional Practice

Health and Interprofessional Practice is a peer-reviewed, open access journal with a focus on publishing high quality evidence of interprofessional practice and education to inform improved patient care. The journal has an international perspective and is published by faculty from Pacific University's College of Health Professions and University Library in collaboration with health professions colleagues at other institutions.

Types of articles published are:
Original theory and research
Case-based learning
Educational strategies
Cross cultural issues in care
Review articles

In addition the journal welcomes articles 'From the Field: Student Experiences'. These are brief descriptive pieces from students reflecting on their experiences of working in multiprofessional teams as a part of their clinical placements. The focus is on what the student has learned about another profession or the challenges/opportunities as a result of their experiences.

The Journal of the Allied Health

The Journal of Allied Health is the official publication of the Association of Schools of Allied Health Professions (ASAHP). The journal's focus is scholarly articles, research and development in the health sector, aligned to a multidisciplinary approach. It is published in the USA but with 30% of subscribers from outside the USA.

Types of published articles are:
Original research
Research notes – for smaller scale studies
Commentary
Potential patterns
Special features

In addition, articles that describe innovative approaches to answering research questions and new approached to data analysis are welcomed under 'Methodological Corner'.

The impact factor is 0.29

Journal of Interprofessional Education and Practice

The *Journal of Interprofessional Education and Practice* is published by Elsevier and is the official journal of the National Academies of Practice (NAP) and affiliated to the University of Nebraska. It is a peer-reviewed online only journal that is published on a quarterly basis. The main focus is on current issues and trends in IP healthcare. It publishes peer-reviewed articles covering a broad range of IP areas of interest. The impact factor is 0.45.

Education for Health

Education for Health (EfH) is a peer-reviewed, free open-access journal produced by The Network: Towards Unity for Health. This is a worldwide consortium of health professions schools committed to enhancing the learning experience of all health professionals to meet the needs of the communities they serve.

The readership of EfH includes a broad range, including policy makers, health care professionals, health care educators and learners.

Types of articles published are:
Original studies
Reviews
Think pieces
Commentary on current trends

Organisations with Major IPE Programmes

Models of Interprofessional Education

In this section reflections on, and descriptions of, institutional models of IPE
will be provided. These are from around the globe reflecting the different but
similar approaches and challenges. The following will be explored:

1 The Linköping IPE model – Sweden
2 MDT FIT- England
3 TeamSTEPPS – USA
4 The Leicester model – England
5 Regional Interprofessional Education (RIPE) – England
6 Curtin University – Australia
7 Minnesota – USA

The Linköping IPE Model

Wilhelmsson et al. (2009) provide a summary of the IPE work undertaken in
Sweden to develop an IPE model.

In 1986, with changes in infrastructure in Sweden, there was an opportunity to develop a fresh approach to undergraduate (UG) training and education across a number of professions. The cornerstone was to enable students
to develop their own professional identity by interaction with other health
and social care professions.

The key themes developed early on remained over a 20-year period. Those
were, early patient contact, communication skills, pre-clinical integration
and clinical integration, scientific rigour, critical thinking and learning
through small group work in the shape of problem-based learning (PBL).

The first initiative was an integrated common module within the first few
weeks on UG programmes across medicine, nursing, occupational therapy,
physiotherapy, medical biology and speech and language pathology. This
comprised 12 weeks experience of a module called 'Man and Society' the
aim of which was to engender common values, common language, critical
thinking, team working and a PBL approach.

In addition, IPE student training wards were introduced. All students across
the professions in their last trimester were as a team jointly responsible for

'running' an orthopaedic ward for two weeks. This was undertaken with expert supervision in place. The aim was for the students, as a team to exercise autonomy, team-based and patient-centred practice.

Around 2000, further revision was precipitated by the presence of new faculty. The previous 'Man and Society' module was reviewed and revised and renamed Health, Ethics and Learning (HEL). The previous 12 weeks was condensed to 8 weeks with a focus on PBL, small group work, problem solving, dealing with conflict and knowledge and language,

In 2003 HEL II was introduced with an additional two weeks module that all students across the professions participated in during years two or three. The focus was sexuality ('Sexology') as a cross-cutting theme with the aim of the students gaining complementary professional competencies, with the use of role-play to learn both with and from one another. Also at this point, the student training wards had been extended to include two orthopaedic and one geriatric ward.

The authors reflected on lessons learnt over a 20 years period which were;

1 the need to have ongoing discussion, evaluation and revision of the IPE offer within the organisation,
2 for success there is a need for IPE educational leadership,
3 for IPE to be embedded requires communication and diplomacy skills,
4 the need to ensure that the IPE learning is relevant to day-to-day practice, ensuring ownership by learners and faculty,
5 involve the learners,
6 involve the faculty, and
7 teaching techniques such as small group work, interactive and clinical problem based learning are essential.

MDT Feedback for Improving Teamwork (FIT)

MDT FIT was developed by Green Cross Medical, funded by the National Cancer Action team (Taylor et al. 2012). Green Cross Medical was established in 2010 with a group of experts in team working with the aim of brining this expertise to practical application to enhance Multidisciplinary Team (MDT) working in the National Health Service (NHS). MDT FIT is designed to enable cancer MDTs to self-assess and obtain feedback on their performance against agreed standards in *The Characteristics of an Effective MDT* (Nation Cancer Action Team 2010). This report described recommendations for effective MDT working under five domains;

1 The team,
2 The infrastructure for meetings,
3 Meeting organisation and logistics,
4 Patient-centred clinical decision-making, and
5 Team governance.

The Team

This is broken down into membership, attendance, leadership, team working and culture, and personal development and training. The membership of the team focuses on the need for all relevant professions and disciplines to be represented with explicit plans to cover absences with deputies and alternatives. There is also a requirement that members of the MDT have the level of expertise and specialism mapped to the nature of the MDT.

In terms of attendance MDT members must have dedicated time within job plans and that the core members are present for the discussion of all cases with a register of attendance taken. The Chair of the MDT is responsible for raising concerns about non-attendance of particular members and escalating these concerns. Regular non-attendance should be fed into the job appraisal and planning.

Within the leadership requirements, there is a need for an identified leader or Chair of the MDT who has clearly articulated roles and responsibilities around the management and logistical operational issues as well as governance.

In terms of team working and culture, the requirements are that each member will have clearly defined roles and responsibilities again included in their job plans, but the team have agreed acceptable team behaviours.

With personal development and training there is a requirement for team members to recognise the need for continuing professional development mapped to those clinical roles and requirements with a need for access to wider training opportunities to meet the roles and responsibilities within an MDT such as leadership, chairing and communication skills.

Infrastructure for Meetings

Within this is physical environment of the meeting venue, technology and equipment.

Physical environment of the meeting venue

There is a requirement for dedicated MDT room in a suitable quiet location so that the necessary confidential discussions can take place. The room must be of an appropriate size and layout so that all team members have a seat.

Technology and Equipment

In terms of technology and equipment the requirement for access to, for example, Picture Archiving and Communication System (PACS) or appropriate databases, video or projection facilities with the requirement for broader technical support for the MDT meeting.

Meeting Organisation and Logistics

Within this there are the areas of scheduling the meetings, preparation prior to meetings, organisation and administration during meetings and post MDT meetings to ensure co-ordination of services.

Scheduling of MDT meetings

The meetings must take place on a regular basis as set out in the Manual of Cancer Services and that the meetings take place during core hours where possible.

Preparation prior to the meetings

That there are processes for deciding cut off time for inclusion of a case to be discussed in the MDT. That the cases are organised on the agenda in a logical sequence and that there is a locally agreed minimum dataset of information about patients to be discussed, pathology radio results, and so on.

Organisation administration

During the meetings there is a requirement that there is clarity in regard to who wants to discuss any particular patient and what the particular issues are. That through the meeting there is access for all of the team members to relevant information in regard to patient notes, sample results, test results, and so on including electronic databases.

In regard to post MDT meeting co-ordination of services there is a requirement that processes are in place for communicating the MDT recommendations to patients, GPs and other clinical teams involved in the patient care and that processes are in place to ensure actions agreed in the meeting are implemented.

Patient-centred Clinical Decision Making

The following areas are covered; Who do discuss? Patient centred care and the clinical decision-making process.

Who to discuss?

There is a requirement for local process to be in place to identify all patients who may require discussion at the MDT and that specific referral criteria are in place with local agreements.

Patient-centred care

There is a requirement that patients are aware of the MDT and its purpose and membership and those patients are aware of when that MDT is and that their case is being discussed. Patients should be informed of the outcome within a locally agreed timeframe. There is also a requirement that the patient's or relative's views are represented by a member of the MDT who has met the patient wherever possible.

Clinical decision-making process

There is a requirement for the MDTs to consider all clinically appropriate treatment options for a given patient, even if these cannot be provided locally. The MDTs have access to a list of all relevant clinical trials and consider each patient's suitability in regard to decision making. There is also a need for a standard treatment protocols and that any clinical decision-making process is evidenced based, for example in line with The National Institute for Health and Care Excellence (NICE) guidelines, patient centred and in line with local protocols.

Team Governance

Within the requirements the following areas are covered, organisational support, data collection analysis and audit outcomes and clinical governance.

Organisational support

There is a requirement for employer support for the MDT meetings which is demonstrated by evidence that the MDTs are an accepted model to deliver safe high-quality care and that the support and funding through job plans, and so on is adequate.

Data collection analysis and audit outcomes

There is a requirement that data collection resources are available to the meeting and that mandatory national data sets or audits are populated prior to or during meetings wherever possible. There is also a need for data collected during MDT meetings to be analysed and fed back to provide other MDTs to support learning. There is also a need for the MDTs to take part in external and internal audits.

Clinical governance

There is a need for agreed policies, guidelines and protocols for operational policy, membership roles and responsibilities. There is a need for user partnership groups to be in existence to advise on the development of MDT policy and practice. There is also a requirement for mechanisms to be in place to record all of the MDT recommendations and compare these to the actual treatment given, particularly if the recommendations are not able to be delivered locally or not adopted for whatever reason and also process to ensure that the MDT is alerted to serious treatment complications or adverse unexpected events/death within the treatment.

In practice, MDT FIT is a web-based platform enabling individual MDTs to complete a process with the aim of obtaining feedback to improve the quality of care to patients. It is a three-stage process usually completed over an 8–12 week period and then revisited on at least an annual basis.

Stage 1 – All MDT members fill in an online survey.

Stage 1b – The survey results are assessed independently together with at least an observational assessment of at least one MDT member.

Stage 2 – The feedback is shared with all MDT members and their MDT FIT facilitator.

Stage 3a – The MDT leader and the facilitator meet to discuss the feedback.

Stage 3b – There is a facilitated MDT discussion with the team agreeing an action plan.

Stage 3c – The facilitator and team leader discuss with the Trust management any changes that require Trust action.

Actions are then implemented, and reviewed in a continuous quality improvement cycle.

In summary, MDT FIT allows cancer MDTs to self-assess against detailed national standards for MDTs, obtain independent feedback, identify and action plan for improvement and ensure these actions are implemented. The aim is to improve service to patients. The unique point with MDT FIT is that the standards are detailed, allowing practical benchmarking. In addition the independent feedback allows the teams to adapt and have ownership of the action plans.

TeamSTEPPS

TeamSTEPPS was developed by the Department of Defense in collaboration with the Agency for Health Care Research and Quality. It is a teamwork and communication system designed to help clinical teams increase their effectiveness in the spheres of communication, leadership, situation monitoring and mutual support.

The aim is to improve patient safety. TeamSTEPPS has been used in a variety of clinical contexts including an Emergency Department (Turner 2012) and Operating Room (Stringer et al. 2015).There are three phases in the programme, initial assessment of the site for readiness, then training for onsite trainers with the last phase the implementation and spread of improvements.

The core of TeamSTEPPS is developing four skills, leadership, situation monitoring, mutual support and communication.

Within this framework there are two types of leaders (i) designated and (ii) situational.

These operate at a very practical level in the clinical setting. Situational monitoring is the process of continually assessing what is happening so that you know what is going on around you. The STEP approach is central...

S ... Status of the patient

T ... Team members

E ... Environment

P ... Progress towards the goal

Within TeamSTEPPS very practical tools in communication are embedded. For example 'CUSS' words are used. These are key phrases that all team members are trained to listen for and react to;

I am Concerned

I am Uncomfortable

This is a Safety issue

I don't feel Safe

The rule is that if any one member of the team voices a 'CUSS' word twice the team must reset or 'stop the line'. Also techniques such as call outs and call backs, the latter is restating what has been asked for, the closed-loop communication.

TeamSTEPPS comprises three phases.

Phase 1 – Assess the Need

The first step is to identify the appropriate MDT with leaders embedded who are committed to change. Then there is a training needs analysis so that the training can be bespoke and tailored to the needs and to the problem or challenges that the team want to address. What should fall out of this process is a list of objectives designed to reduce risk to patients. Each objective is described in one simple sentence … what will be achieved, who will do what, when and how.

Phase 2 – Planning, Training and Implementation

A detailed training plan is designed, targeting certain individuals or a more whole-team training. An implementation plan of the training is then detailed and proposed to leaders of the organisation. Once the plan is agreed it is important to communicate the plan with the focus on the outcome of patient safety. The change team have to work within the work environment to set the conditions whereby change can occur. The training is then implemented and can consist of:

A two day training course to train the trainer; and

TeamSTEPPS fundamental – six 6 hour sessions of interactive workshops

Phase 3 – Sustaining the TeamSTEPPS Intervention

In this phase there are a number of steps described to ensure that change is embedded and sustained, including providing opportunities for the team to practice their new skills.

Leaders must lead the change and facilitate team engagement in the ongoing continuous improvement process. In this continuous improvement cycle, it is important to quantify success. Data are important to show that the desired changes in process and patient outcomes have been achieved and these successes need to celebrated.

The Leicester Model

The Leicester IPE model began in 1995 with the recognition of the need for medical students to understand the multiprofessional and multiagency context of care delivery. There have been a range of publications that describe the evolution of this model (Anderson and Lennox 2009; Anderson et al. 2016).

From the beginning of this model, a key principle was immersion of the leaners at the front line of service delivery in primary care.

The programme began as a 2-day course and over a 10-year period has developed to now include 8 professions with student numbers involved reported in the academic year 2017–2018 in excess of 900. The Leicester model describes four stages of learning beginning with immersion of the learners into patientcare and professional experiences. Students of mixed professions are allocated to a number of primary care sites, local health centres or community facilities. Students work in small groups of four and begin by interviewing a patient whose journey they 'follow'. The interview typically takes place in the patient's home with the purpose of the students as a team assessing the impact of a number of issues on the patient's wellbeing. The student team then interview the health care practitioners involved in delivering care to their patient to explore the strengths and weaknesses of the service provision for that patient. They then reflect with a tutor/facilitator and then present to the local delivery team and discuss ways in which care could be improved thus completing the learning cycle.

Lessons learnt from decades of the Leicester model (Anderson et al. 2016) include:

1 Successful IPE can only develop over time. A key tactic is to commence small and evolve. This approach echoes with the principles underpinning a Plan Do Study Act (PDSA) quality improvement cycle with small multiple steps (see Chapter 2 definitions).
2 There is a need to engage with patients/carers, the clinical delivery teams and the learners.
3 Shared partnership at the organisational level is essential. This is typically across Higher Education Institution, NHS and social care and including the third sector. High-level strategic agreement is needed and this in turn allows the development of joint working at the coalface level, for example sharing space and resources.
4 A key element is ensuring the practice practitioners are trained in the IPE process, not just a one off but an ongoing programme of support and continuing professional development.

The unique aspect of the Leicester model is the immersion of a small team of different professions following and reflecting on the individual patient's experience.

Regional Interprofessional Education (RIPE) Project

This project is a part of the NHS Executive South West Region in England drive to quality improvement with a focus on patient scare (Hinds and Todres 2002). There are many examples of different projects but one example used to give a flavour of the processes and wider advantages is the 'Castlebury Experience'. This is a rural town with a District General Hospital. The focus of this project was on three wards providing care to older people.

The clinical team was formed into an action learning group (ALG) supported by a team from Bournemouth University (BU). The ALG at the initial stages comprised:

> physiotherapist, ward sister/clinical nurse specialist, occupational therapist, consultant in old age care and then a social services professional joined to make a multiprofessional cross agencies team. The BU team comprised a Continuous Quality Improvement (CQI) facilitator, lecturer practitioner (with nurse educator background) and an educator with a social worker background.

The aim was to lead to improvement in health outcomes for patients and to provide pre- and post-qualification IP learning experiences.

The PDSA cycle (see Chapter 2 definitions) was used as the process to achieve continuous improvement. After initial meetings of the ALG the specific QI 'niggle' identified was the number of inappropriate re-admissions. There was then a series of meetings working through the 'problem', as a team with support from the BU team. There were several cycles of test and retesting changes in process in the care pathway including, in particular, knowledge handling and pre-discharge planning. This cycle of feedback led to refinement in processes with agreement to use the unified Kardex system as the focal point for patient information and hence the basis for care planning.

This was an example of the PDSA in action in a real clinical setting with a team approach supported by outside 'expert' educational/process improvement intervention.

The unique selling point with this example is the embedding of a small education team within a small service delivery team.

Curtin University, Western Australia

Brewer and Barr (2016) describe the developments in Curtin University, Western Australia. This team-based IP practice placement (TIPP) began in 2009 with five small pilots. In 2016 the university provided TIPP to over 500 students across nine health and social care professions.

Curtin University in Perth Western Australia had approximately 11 000 students in seven health schools: nursing, midwifery, and paramedic medicine; occupational therapy and social work; psychology and speech pathology: pharmacy; biomedical sciences; public health; physiotherapy and exercise science.

The initial change was the introduction of case-based workshops by a number of champions. This quickly evolved into the five pilot TIPPs for groups of two to five professionals, four in community-based services and one in the university.

Today Curtin University works to an IPE framework based on:

Client-centred service;

Client safety and quality; and

Collaborative practice

A range of practice-based IP clinical placements are available. One example is the Cockburn Integrated Health and Community facility, located in Success and opened in 2104. The service is focused on providing client-centred care to the local community with an emphasis on the management of chronic conditions, for example diabetes, chronic pain and rheumatoid arthritis. The services are delivered by students, under supervision of qualified staff, across a range of professions, speech pathology, occupational therapy, physiotherapy, social work and nursing. The students get involved in initial interprofessional screening of clients, goal setting, and the development of a care plan.

Lessons learnt included:

1 At an organisational level it is important to choose partners wisely. TIPP will be more successful or have more chance of success if all partners are committed to preparing graduates for the future.

2 The HEI to practice placement must be mutually beneficial and it is important to have formal agreements in place at both strategic and operational levels.

3 Build in evaluation and continuous quality improvement from the beginning.

4 Learners need time to consolidate learning, so placement should be a minimum of two weeks full time or equivalent.

5 The timing of the TIPP it is argued is optimal nearer the end of their UG education when learners have already developed a clearer sense of their own professional identity.

Minnesota

In the USA, there is one model that has had a major impact on IPE and health care delivery. In 2012, the National Centre for Interprofessional Practice and Education was launched at the University of Minnesota. It has quickly established itself as a vibrant hub supporting a community of practice of IPE across many states in the USA. The centre is referred to as the *The Nexus,* and its focus is on building and enhancing partnerships between health professions education and health care providers.

The Nexus has partnered with a wide range of academic health organisations to collate all data from large-scale IPE trials into a national data repository. The aim of this big database is to demonstrate and share the impact of team-based health care on patients. This platform also acts as a facilitator for virtual communities of practice with functions to allow discussions, sharing experiences and asking questions.

An important driver for change has been the formation of the Interprofessional Education Collaborative (IPEC) and the development of the IPEC competencies. These competencies have been used to drive change in health-related curricula facilitating change across a network in the USA.

The centre uses a range of tools including the Stairstep Model as a tool for teams embarking on or refreshing IPC projects/initiatives to use to realise their vision.

The Stairstep model describes a sequence of activities that facilitate the goal of integrated health care and higher education system transformation resulting in improved health and learning outcomes.

For multiprofessional teams the sequence of steps are;

Step 1. Getting to know each other
The key tasks in this step are to convene key stakeholders together to get to know each other prior to any IPE activity.

Step 2. Teamwork
The need for a planned educational/training on teamwork, knowledge, skills and behaviours including values.

Step 3. Patient safety/quality
The planned use of IPE to learn about the patient and address patient safety and quality issues.

Step 4. Access to care
The planned use of IPE as a method to improve patients' access to care.

Step 5. Workforce optimisation
The key tasks include moving from teaching to the emphasis being on learning and in a particular learning in the workplace. Incorporate IPE into the processes for redesign and modernisation of the workforce.

Step 6. Health outcomes
Explicitly make a link between IPE and improvements to all levels of health outcomes.

Step 7. Driving cost out of the system
Plan to develop and implement IPE models that are designed to lower health costs and also lower costs in health education.

Chapter Summary

There is a wide range of organisations across the world that champion IPE and related collaborative practice. In addition, there are journal publications with a specific focus on IPE and an increasing realisation from mainstream journals that IPE is increasingly important.

Across the world, there are examples of 'movements' and specific institutions that have championed IPE and led to a growing community of practice in IPE and collaborative practice. The common lessons learnt include: learner engagement, faculty engagement, collaboration between health and social care providers, and that innovation sometimes requires small steps at a time.

References

Anderson, S.E., Ford, J., and Kinnair, D. (2016). Interprofessional education and practice guide no. 6: developing practice-based interprofessional learning using short placement model. *Journal of Interprofessional Care* 30 (4): 433–440.

Anderson, E.S. and Lennox, A. (2009). The Leicester model of interprofessional education: developing, delivering and learning from student voices for 10 years. *Journal of Interprofessional Care* 23 (6): 557–573.

Brewer, M.L. and Barr, H. (2016). Interprofessional education and practice guide no. 8: team-based interprofessional practice placements. *Journal of Interprofessional Education* 30 (6): 747–753.

Hindes, D. and Todres, L. (2002). *The RIPE Project: A Regional Interprofessional Education Project Co-ordinated by Bournemouth University*. Bournemouth, UK: Bournemouth University.

National Cancer Action Team. (2010). The characteristics of an effective multidisciplinary team. London; National Cancer Action Team. www.ncin.org.uk/mdt. (accessed: 30 June 2018).

Nisbet, G., Thistlethwaite, J., Chesters, J. et al. (2007). Sharing a vision for collaborative practice: the formation of an Australasian interprofessional practice and education network (AIPPEN). *Focus on Health Professional Education* 8 (3): 1–7.

Stringer, M., Weld, L., Ebertowski, J. et al. (2015). Team strategies and tools to enhance performance and patient safety (Team STEPPS) improves operating room efficiency. *The Journal of Urology* 193 (4S): e168.

Taylor, C., Brown, K., Lamb, B. et al. (2012). Developing and testing TEAM (Team Evaluation and Assessment Measure), a self-assessment tool to improve cancer multidisciplinary teamwork. *Annals of Surgical Oncology* 19: 4019–4027.

Turner, P. (2012). Implementation of the TeamSTEPPS in the emergency department. *Critical Care Nursing Quarterly* 35 (3): 208–212.

Wilhelmsson, M., Pelling, S., Ludvigsson, J. et al. (2009). Twenty years experience of interprofessional education in Linköping – ground-breaking and sustainable. *Journal of Interprofessional Care* 23 (2): 121–133.

Chapter 6 **Evaluation of Interprofessional Education**

Introduction

This chapter will explore the principles, challenges, and possible solutions to the development of effective assessment strategies for Interprofessional Education (IPE). A range of different approaches to and levels of assessment of IPE will be explored and critically analysed.

One regular criticism of the published evaluations of IPE-type educational interventions, explored in Chapter 3, is that the specific teaching strategies used are not described. This makes it difficult to ascertain what level if any the interventions were at. A regular theme is team training which has a number of definitions (see Chapter 2). Some of the specific approaches used, for example the PRECEDE/PROCEED model and the Theory of Planned Behaviour, do not readily align with the published work on what constitutes IPE.

There are a number of fundamental questions that need to be addressed in regard to the assessment of IPE interventions. The key question remains unanswered; what are the core characteristics that define an IPE educational intervention and which specific aspects are effective in achieving the changes required?

The studies described in Chapter 3, as examples, show a diverse range of outcomes. Barceló et al. (2010) using the Plan Do Study Act (PDSA) cycle, showed a statistically significantly improvement in blood glucose control. Neither the educational strategy or the professional profiles of learners are clearly described. Thompson et al. (1998) found an improved level of asking about domestic violence in a primary care setting. They used the PRECEDE/ PROCEED model, usually used in change-management programmes. The educational strategies did describe interaction as a key element with an explicit objective of each participant understanding each other's roles.

How to Succeed at Interprofessional Education, First Edition. Peter Donnelly.
© 2019 John Wiley & Sons Ltd. Published 2019 by John Wiley & Sons Ltd.

These two examples highlight the heterogeneity of the educational interventions that make it difficult to draw general conclusions of the effects of particular aspects of the IPE experience.

So the starting point is how do we identify the key elements that make an IPE intervention truly interprofessional? Harden provided a three dimensional model almost 20 years ago and although it is a useful there has been no practical tool until Xyrichis and colleagues described a framework in 2017. This may turn out to be a practical tool for researchers and educators to use to identify at what level their education interventions lie.

When considering any evaluation of education/training the following questions need to asked and answered to help shape the methodology for the study:

What is my research question?

What do I what to measure?

How will I show change?

At what level do I wish to show change?

At what level can I expect change to be shown?

Is this at an individual, team, patient or system level?

Specifically for IPE evaluations the following are useful areas to consider:

1 the context in which the IPE is to be used;
2 the expected learning objectives;
3 the specific teaching strategies along the IPE continuum that are to be used. Specific reference to an agreed framework would enable any study to be replicated and or compared to similar work.

General Principles of Evaluation

The design principles of IPE educational initiatives are covered in Chapter 4. In this section, the general principles of evaluation are considered. In addition, practical considerations are explored to help in the planning of the evaluation process. The following areas will be discussed:

1 The initial steps
2 The scope
3 Types of evaluation
4 Ethical issues
5 Access to data
6 Resources for evaluation
7 Techniques for data gathering
8 Commonly used theories/models
9 Conducting the evaluation
10 Dissemination strategy

The Initial Steps

When considering evaluating any educational activity there are initial basic questions to be answered. Why undertake the assessment? What is the key question that needs answered? What is the overall aim of the evaluation? For example, is it to test a hypothesis that a specific teaching technique, such as case-based small group work with nurses and pharmacists improves case identification of hypertension?

There can be more specific reasons for evaluating educational initiatives and these include:

1 Measuring achievement of specific learning outcomes and or aims. The latter can be specific obligations or aims expected by a health education commissioner.
2 To help to inform decision-making in regard to resources allocation. This is particularly important in today's financial environment where scarce financial and other resources need to be redirected to where they can achieve more value for the resources invested. This reflects back to one of the Triple Aims of achieving value and financial sustainability (Berwick et al. 2008).
3 Evaluation can be used to compare and contrast different educational approaches or to compare different types of approaches within IPE.
4 To test the effectiveness of learning in one particular multiprofessional setting in a scientific manner so that the approach can be compared against other sectors.

Hence, there may be a range of reasons one might undertake evaluation of educational initiatives within an IPE setting and it is essential to be clear in terms of the general aims and specific objectives of embarking on such an evaluation.

The Scope

The next step is to agree the scope of the evaluation. This is essentially a statement of what the evaluation will and will not cover. This is an important early step that will reduce the risk of the aims not being met and that scope creep does not occur. This is the scenario whereby the study expands to include aspects that were not planned for and therefore may not be deliverable. The scope also helps in defining the methodology used within the evaluation itself.

There are a number of key questions that can help in deciding the scope of the evaluation and this is similar to any research work, that is, what the research question is. Some key questions include:

- What do you want to evaluate and why?
- How would answering these questions contribute to meeting the needs of internal and external stakeholders?

- How should the evaluation be conducted? Based on the methodology what skill set is going to be needed?
- When will the evaluation begin? How long will it last?

Before commencing it is important to understand any constraints and barriers there may be in relation to the type of methodology of evaluation proposed.

In terms of the research question, it is useful to know what data are already readily available within the environment to be studied. Sometimes it is appropriate to ask the question that requires generation of new processes to gather the data. It is however important in the initial planning stages to explore what sources of data are already there. It is so much easier to use already existing and validated sources of data, such as national audits.

Types of Evaluation

In general terms evaluation of educational initiatives undertaken are most often under the categories of formative or summative. It is best to see these two constructs as lying along a continuum. At one end of the spectrum, formative assessment is used as a tool to help learners guide their own learning. It aims to provide detailed feedback for each learning encounter to allow learners to reflect on and enhance their own learning.

At the other end of the continuum is summative assessment used to observe a change in the learners' behaviour so that a judgement can be made as to whether they have achieved the relevant learning objectives.

In general terms, within the educational community, the distinction between formative and summative has become blurred in recent years. The distinction between them is less important and in fact most evaluations will be of a hybrid nature which essentially means containing formative and summative elements.

Other types of investigation include interpretive or descriptive or more commonly a mixed-method approach which essentially combines qualitative and quantitative approaches. Quantitative data can take the form of questionnaires with specific data included for example, scores on the Likert scale combined with the qualitative data from for example, semi-structured interviews or focus groups. So, the results in these mixed-method studies take the form of statistical analysis of the quantitative data and a narrative descriptive report of the qualitative data.

Another approach is the experimental evaluation and examples of this are covered in Chapter 3, particularly in terms of randomised controlled trials, controlled before and after and time-interrupted studies.

Ethical Issues

As a general principle, it is extremely important to ensure there is adequate ethical consideration of any evaluation. This is particularly important as within educational interventions individual human beings or groups of human beings are usually subject to participation in the study, that is, it is a human-subjects-based research and as such it is important to consider ethical issues.

It is also equally important to consider the contractual arrangements of any participants within the study. For example, in the United Kingdom, community pharmacists may be independent contractors and on the other hand, advanced nurse practitioners on acute medical wards will be NHS employees. In a study involving these two professions due consideration has to be given to the governance and to human resources arrangements for those potential participants in any study.

It is important to understand the context in which the participants and the learning takes place so therefore it is important to understand the details of the local context. Prior to embarking on any formal evaluation, information gathering at a pre-research stage can be extremely important. This can take the form of informal conversations with internal stakeholders. These preliminary explorations can used to sense check any specific aims and objectives you might have for the educational initiative and to explore the reality of any constraints or barriers that may be present. It is clear that those individuals closest to the delivery of the continuous professional development are likely to be best placed to understand these.

It is also important to understand the wider context of any educational initiative and therefore it is important again, depending on the scope and breadth of what is being proposed, to undertake at least a light literature review if not a systematic review following examples such as the Cochrane Reviews. The latter are considered to be the highest standard in evidenced-based health care.

Access to Data

Most studies evaluating IPE initiatives will require gathering data from a range of professionals and patients. It is important when embarking to consider the breadth and scope to make sure that one has access to the participants and in particular the patients. This goes back to the ethical considerations in regards to access to patient notes, data collection and one has to be very cognisant of the General Data Protection Regulation that came into force in May 2018. This gives the individual more control in how their personal data are handled.

It is extremely important once the scope and breadth have been decided to commence describing the details of the evaluation plan. Because of the inevitable complex nature of the evaluation of educational initiatives in a health care setting it is important that this plan is a live document and reviewed and revised in light of any changes or difficulties that may arise. One of the key elements to the plan has to be to describe the methodology in clear terms. Some key elements to consider in the methodology are;

Explain the rationale for using the methods including the context.

How data were gathered, what specific tools or techniques were used?

Was the sample large enough?

How was the sample selected?

How was the data obtained, processed and then analysed?

Was statistical analysis used and/or was a specific theoretical framework used to explain observed behaviours?

Describe the potential limitations to the methods.

Resources for Evaluation

As touched on earlier it is important to be clear from the beginning, that is, in the pre-planning stages the totality of the resources required in order to answer the research question. From the very beginning, it is important to describe any potential costs which can include the following:

1 The need for external statistical analysis and interpretation.

2 Purchase of recording equipment or software to help support analysis of data.

3 Staffing costs in regard to interviewers or online developers for online questionnaires or web app development.

4 Administration costs; photocopying, printing, developing a website.

With most educational evaluations the most expensive single item is staff time. This is why it important to pre-plan and one option is to use a Gantt chart (Gantt 1910). This is essentially a bar chart that is used to describe a project plan. The horizontal axis represents the total time span of the project broken down into intervals, hours, days, months, and so on depending on the projected time frame or deadlines. The vertical axis represents the separate tasks that are required to complete the project. Gantt charts provide a quick visual illustration of the status of any project. There are a number of types and formats that can be used and all are available online.

One issue with Gantt charts is that they do not readily illustrate interdependencies and one alternative option is to use the PERT (Program Evaluation Review Technique) chart.

If using a mixed-method study, for example semi-structured interviews, the most expensive elements are likely to be the interviewers' time to analyse the code and the transcripts from the interviews. This is likely to involve the use of a software package, such as NVIVO10. This is a qualitative data analysis software package that is extremely useful in analysing text-rich data such as transcriptions from semi-structured interviews. NVIVO allows the downloading of a range of documents such as Microsoft Word, PDFs, audio files, and files from the IBM SPSS Statistics package. The software allows automated analysis of text-rich data using a range of theoretical models such as grounded theory, ethnography and mixed methods. These and other methods are described briefly later as all of these can be used to evaluate any learning and hence are appropriate for IPE evaluations.

Techniques for Data Gathering
Common data gathering techniques for qualitative research include;
Surveys
Semi-structured interviews
Focus groups
These will be described briefly for completeness.

Surveys
Online surveys or questionnaires are a useful tool in qualitative research. There are a number of key rules for their design. There is a logical sequence to constructing a questionnaire. The first is to be clear about the research question and this needs to be informed by published work in the area, to help ensure a good response that your main research question is meaningful to potential respondents.

Knowledge of the target population is essential in designing the questionnaire as is the format, balance of open and closed questions and the level at which to pitch the questions.

Before considering the construction of individual items it is important to consider the formatting of the questionnaire, how it is laid out, organised and presented. The formatting will have an impact on how easy it is to complete and hence improve the response rate (Bradburn et al. 2004).

The questionnaire needs to take into account the motivation of potential respondents. The response rate is improved if the questionnaire is perceived as an opportunity for the respondents to voice their concerns and their views with the possibility of influencing change (Ekeh 1974).

In terms of the items, there are a number of key issues to take into consideration.

The first question should be general but directly linked to the aim of the questionnaire. It should be applicable to all respondents and be simple and easy to understand.

The ordering of questions and any groupings of questions needs to be considered. Logical ordering helps the flow of the questionnaire (Babbie 1973). The manner in which respondents answer questions is significantly influenced by cognitive and normative processes. For example, a respondent's answer to a question will be influenced by the answer to the previous question, the 'anchoring effect'. Following a very negative response to one question, the respondent may attempt to balance their responses with a highly positive answer to the next question, the 'subtraction effect' (Dillman 2000).

Keeping the language simple is important, for example do not use double negatives. Each question should address one single issue or idea. It is best to avoid double questions – questions with two or more unrelated parts – as these are difficult to answer.

There needs to be a balance between open and closed questions. Open questions allow the respondent to expand and it is useful to offer the opportunity to do so. On the other hand they can be difficult to answer and the answers may be a challenge to code and analyse.

It is best to avoid using vague ill-defined terms ... such as ... 'do middle age people cough more?' How does one define middle age? This will mean different things to different people.

It is important to remember that not all respondents will have a view, or that each question is applicable to all so include, *don't know* or *not applicable* as options. In addition, it is best to avoid the use of jargon or abbreviations – do not assume everyone will understand.

For more complex questionnaires the navigation pathway is important. This relates to how the questionnaire branches out depending on the respondent's answers. The use of clear visual clues such as symbols can aid navigation (Redline and Dillman 2002).

Iglesias and Torgerson (2000) showed that the length of the questionnaire is an important factor in response rates with a significant difference in response rate between short and long questionnaires.

Interviews
Interviews allow in-depth and detailed exploration of the subject area and can also give more accurate insights to respondents' attitudes, thoughts and actions. This methodology can be used to explore novel areas for further research. The interview approach may uncover previously unconsidered issues. In a semi-structured approach the interviewer typically begins with a number of open-ended questions and then probes participants' responses, encouraging them to provide detail and clarification.

A hybrid of self-completion questionnaires and interviews (so called 'questerviews' have been described (Adamson et al. 2004) and this multimethod technique is advocated in health related research.

Disadvantages to interviews includes the fact they are labour intensive, and hence costly, so invariably the number of respondents is restricted but the response rate is higher than with an online approach.

Similar to any human interaction, interviewer bias can be a factor. The interviewer can potentially influence the interviewee, via the framing of questions and non-verbal communication. Examples include, asking leading questions, selective attendance to responses, over or under identification with the interviewees and misinterpretation. This can be mitigated to a certain extent by ensuring that the evaluators/ interviewers have undergone standardised training and there is a sampling of the interviewers' interactions in terms of benchmarking against standards so that one avoids the risk of one or two interviewers differentially affecting participants' responses.

It is important to have a sampling method that ensures everyone in the target population has an equal chance of being selected. This will remove a level of bias. The best option to achieve this is a randomised sample so that one can extrapolate statistically from the sample to the population being studied. In qualitative studies, sampling becomes important as a tool to remove the bias of the researcher in picking whom to interview; it becomes essential in ensuring replicable results and needed to ensure accuracy and validity of responses. On the other hand an advantage to interviews is that due to the presence of the interviewer questions can be explained and or clarified but in doing so further bias can be introduced.

Focus Groups

Focus groups are a widely used technique for gathering qualitative data. They consist of small group of participants, normally 8–10, with a facilitator for the purpose of exploring a specific issue or question. The output includes beliefs and preferences in regard to the issue at hand. There are many types of focus groups that be used depending on the anticipated outcome. Dual facilitated focus groups have two facilitators, one to ask the questions and the other to ensure the smooth running of the process. A focus group with duelling facilitators, is where one each takes an opposing stance in the issue in question acting as 'the devil's advocate' to stimulate discussion. Outputs from focus groups can be noted or the discussion transcribed and analysed using appropriate software (see NVIVO discussed earlier).

Commonly Used Theories/Models

There is a range of theories and models that can be used to underpin the evaluation process and some commonly used approached are discussed briefly. These include;
Grounded theory
Conversation analysis

Ethnography
Phenomenological analysis

Grounded Theory

The premise of grounded theory (Glaser and Strauss 1967) is to generate the theory from the data. The researcher begins with no pre-conceived theory, hypothesis or expectations but allows the theory to emerge from the data. The theory is, therefore, 'grounded' in the data.

Grounded theory is ideal for exploring social relationships and the behaviour of groups where there is little previously published work on the factors (the social processes) that affect the individual's lives. There is a wide range of versions of grounded theory but all have the following features in common;
Simultaneous collection and analysis of data;
Using the data to generate codes, categories and themes;
Using the data to uncover social processes;
Initially constructing abstract categories;
Further data collection to refine those categories; and
The integration of categories into a theoretical model.

This approach typically uses in-depth interviews with open questions initially then these are refined as the theory emerges. Once this happens, further rounds of interviews or focus groups can be used.

Conversation Analysis

Conversation analysis (CA) is a commonly used approach to studying and understanding social interactions. It focuses on both verbal and nonverbal aspects. CA began in the 1960s based on ethnomethodology (Garfinkel 1967). The analysis of conversation is based in the observation of a set of natural structures within any verbal interaction, such as taking turns to speak. This turn taking leads to and builds up a sequence of exchanges of social interactions.

Ethnography

Ethnography developed from anthropological studies of remote societies in the early 1900s when researchers embedded themselves in those societies over long periods of time (Hammersly and Atkinson 1983). In essence, the researchers made in-depth observations of the culture, practice and perceptions of the society. So ethnography is based on observation.

Unlike grounded theory, this approach does begin with pre-conceived hypotheses that are then tested against the observed data. The method is typically to work with unstructured data from a relatively small number of cases. The analysis of the data involves interpretation of the observed factors and the output takes the form generally of narratives and descriptive reports.

Phenomenological Analysis

The basis of the interpretive phenomenological analysis (IPA) approach is to understand how individuals make sense of a given phenomenon (an event, a belief) in certain contexts. Prior assumptions or hypotheses are not made and this approach argues that it is possible to interpret events in many ways depending on the individual's frame of reference. The focus of IPA can be one individual or a small group. It was developed from the original ideas of phenomenology and hermeneutics (Smith 2007). With this approach, in-depth interviews are commonly used to gather data.

Conducting the Evaluation

It can be extremely useful, particularly if using a methodology that the staff haven't used previously, to undertake a test or pilot of that methodology. This can help to identify any constraints or barriers that possibly one is not aware of.

It is important when selecting individuals to lead an evaluation to ensure that they have, if at all possible, an immediate level of credibility with participants and the organisations in which those participants work.

With any study particularly around the quantitative methodology it important to collect baseline data prior to the introduction of the educational initiative and for that baseline data to have a validity mapped to the research questions.

The design of the study must include a process to test validity and reliability.

In its simplest form validity is defined as the extent to which a tool measures what it claims or is designed to measure. There are a number of types of validity:

Content validity – the degree to which the content of a test maps or correlates with the expert view of that construct or subject area.

Concurrent validity – the degree to which results on one test correlate with results of another test/tool designed to measure the same construct.

Predictive validity – the degree to which a test can predict outcomes in the future.

Reliability is defined as the consistency of a measure. High reliability is when similar results are obtained when the 'test' is administered in similar conditions. Types of reliability include:

Inter-rater reliability – the degree to which two or more raters agree on scores when the test is applied at one point in time.

Test-retest reliability – the degree of consistency of test scores between different applications of the test over time.

Dissemination Strategy

At the preplanning stage it is important to agree the dissemination strategy for the results of any study. This will in part be determined by the aims and objectives of the evaluation. This can take many forms from a simple briefing to a more detailed report, to seeking to publish within health and social care education journals such as the *Journal of Interprofessional Care* (see Chapter 5 for IPE-focused journals).

It is also important to consider again at the pre-planning stage dissemination through specific education and health related conferences. These conferences are frequently sponsored and supported by organisations that promote IPE and are described in Chapter 5.

Assessment Tools used in IPE

Before going on to explore some of the evaluation tools both specific to IPE and more generic, for example team working, it is important to understand the context of the IP learning or IP practice learning (IPPL).

Barr and Brewer (2012) described three IPPL placements models and this is a useful framework to consider one's own learning/teaching when embarking on evaluation.

1 The first model is where learners are expected to search out and find IPPL experiences themselves. This may be supported by tutors or trainers.
2 The second model uses the fact that learners are co-located, say on the same campus for different courses, similar to opportunistic learning.
3 The third model is where there is planned and programmed learning opportunities across a number of professions to learn together. Each undertakes the 'usual' activities/tasks of their own profession but in the context of a team providing a patient-centred service.

Although these are just general descriptions, they can be useful to consider when formulating any evaluation questions.

Core Competencies for IPC Practice

There has been an increasing demand for IP educational experiences across a number of professions. For example from the Annual Medical School Questionnaire in the USA, Barzansky and Etzel (2015) reported an increase in medical schools reporting the need for IPE experience from 76 to 92% between 2011 and 2014.

In 2009 in the USA six national associations for health related schools formed a collaborative with the aim of promoting all aspects of IPE. A part of this work involved an expert panel devising a set of core competencies for IPE – the IP Collaborative Practice – that was revised and published in 2016 (Interprofessional Education Collaborative 2016). The aim was to define IPP competencies that would help steer and direct curricula.

In the revised 2016 version, the overarching domain is Interprofessional Collaboration with four core general competencies within this. The core competencies are:

Values and ethics for interprofessional practice;
Roles and responsibilities for collaborative practice;
Interprofessional team work and team-based practice; and
Interprofessional communication practices.

Within each core competency, there are a number of sub-competencies so for example under 'values and ethics for IP practice' there are 10 the first 3 of which are:

> VE 1. *Place interests of patients and populations at the center of inter-professional health care delivery and population health programs and policies, with the goal of promoting health and health equity across the life span.*
> VE 2. *Respect the dignity and privacy of patients while maintaining confidentiality in the delivery of team-based care.*
> VE3. *Embrace the cultural diversity and individual differences that characterize patients, populations, and the health team.*
>
> (Interprofessional Education Collaborative 2016, p. 11)

The earlier version of the IPEC competency domains were used in part as the basis for the development of an IP Attitudes Scale (described later).

Current Evaluation Tools for IPE

These are a range of validated instruments designed specifically for the evaluation of IPE. These include the following:

1 Interdisciplinary education perception scale
2 Readiness for IP learning scale
3 Interprofessional Attitudes Scale
4 Role perception questionnaire
5 Attitudes to Health Professionals Questionnaire
6 University of the West of England IP Questionnaire
7 Interprofessional Education Collaborative Assessment Tool

Interdisciplinary Education Perception Scale

Luecht et al. (1990) reported the development of one of the earliest examples of a questionnaire designed specifically to measure outcomes of interdisciplinary education. The Interdisciplinary Education Perception Scale (IEPS) is an 18 item questionnaire using a Likert type scale, with the purpose of measuring learners' changes in attitude following practice-based IPE. The IEPS is constructed around four factors; professional competency and autonomy;

perceived needs for collaboration; perception of actual co-operation and the value and contributions of other professionals/ professions.

The original factors were devised by an expert group and validated with a sample of 143 participants across occupational therapy (60% of the sample), medical records, speech pathology and audiology and therapeutic recreation.

The IEPS was used by Hayward et al. (1996) to evaluate students' professional perceptions of interdisciplinary practice. The evaluation used a pre- and post-test methodology to explore whether exposure of students to an interdisciplinary care process in a rural setting changed the participants attitudes to interdisciplinary practice. The students (n = 59) were from 10 academic institutions across 5 US states and included nursing, medicine, social work, counselling and physical therapy. The educational intervention was designed to educate students to provide a co-ordinated, effective, co-operative and high quality approach to patient care in a rural setting.

Statistically significant improvements in attitudes pre- and post-test were shown.

The IPES has been widely used with different professional groups including paramedic undergraduates (Williams and Webb 2012) and medical students (Zanotti et al. 2015).

Readiness for IP Learning Scale

The readiness for IP learning scale (RIPLS) was developed as a tool to assess the readiness of health care students for IP learning (Parsell and Bligh 1999). The authors considered that there were a number of conditions and characteristics needed for successful IP learning these were distilled to four key dimensions:

1 the relationship between different professionals;
2 collaboration and team work;
3 roles and responsibilities; and
4 benefits to patients.

The authors devised a pilot questionnaire generated by a review of the literature, interviews with clinicians and academics.

The items in the questionnaire were rated by 13 experts of different professions. The revised questionnaire was them piloted with second year health care students (n = 120) from medicine, dentistry, orthoptists, radiographers, occupational therapy and nursing.

From this, they developed 19 statements arranged in 3 subscales;

1 team-work and collaboration
2 professional identity
3 roles and responsibilities

An example of a statement is;

shared learning with other health care students will increase my ability to understand clinical problems. (Parsell and Bligh 1999, p. 98)

The authors suggest that this tool can be used to explore differences in students' perceptions about IP learning.

McFadyen et al. (2005) undertook further exploration of the original 19 items and described 4 sub-scales which appeared to be a better fit.

The RIPLS was used by Horsburgh et al. (2001) to measure the attitude of first-year medical, nursing and pharmacy students to IPE. The location was the University of Auckland, New Zealand. The students (n = 180) were surveyed at the beginning of their studies. The results were positive in that all groups reported positives attitudes to team working, seen as beneficial to patient care. Nursing and pharmacy students however indicated more strongly that an outcome of learning together would be better team working. Medical students were less certain of their professional identity and reported considering that they need to acquire more knowledge and skills than nursing or pharmacy students do.

Hind et al. (2003) used the RIPLS as a part of wider study with the aim of increasing understanding of students' attitudes towards their own and other professional groups when starting their studies. The location was Kings College London, UK. A total of 933 students were surveyed from medicine, nursing, dietetics, pharmacy and physiotherapy. The overall readiness for IPL was similar in each profession. Further analysis showed that nursing students had slightly higher readiness scores than the other professions.

So, RIPLS has been shown to be a useful and reliable tool for assess readiness of learners for IPL.

Interprofessional Attitudes Scale (IPAS)

The Interprofessional Attitudes Scale (IPAS) developed by Norris et al. (2015) is a tool to measure IP attitudes of health students, based on the IPEC competency domains.

The tool was developed in the University of Utah, Health Sciences Centre. A survey was developed based on two aspects. The first was 26 items based on the extended RIPLS and the second was 16 further new items covering the IPEC competency domains. Each was scored using a five point Likert scale (1 = strongly disagree and 5 = strongly agree).

The survey was administered to over 1500 students covering a wide range of professions, physical therapy, nutrition, postgraduate and undergraduate nursing, pharmacy, medical laboratory sciences, medical doctors, physician associates and public health. After exploratory and factor analysis a 27-item scale with 5 subscales was produced. The five subscales, and an example statement in the first three are:

Team work, roles responsibilities

1.1   Sharing learning before graduation will help me become a better team worker

Patient centeredness

2.1   Establishing trust with my patients is important to me

Interprofessional Biases

3.2   I have prejudices or make assumptions about health professions/ students from other disciplines

Diversity and ethics

Community centeredness

The IPAS has been used across a number of professions. One example is a two-year study of pharmacy trainees which showed that after a 30 hours IP educational intervention trainees showed significant increases in feeling better able to work in IP teams and valued IPP more (Boland et al. 2018).

Role Perception Questionnaire

Mackay (2004) used the repertory grid technique (Kelly 1955) based on the personal construct theory to identify constructs and then developed a role perception questionnaire (RPQ).

The methodology comprised interviews with 16 third year students from eight professional groups, nursing, midwifery, physiotherapy, podiatry, occupational therapy, prosthetics and orthodontics, radiography and social work in the University of Salford, Salford, UK. This generated a pool of 31 bipolar constructs from the students. An example of one is:

Medical focus to work   Social focus to the work

Further analysis identified the 20 most popular with the final questionnaire scoring these on a linear scale 1–10.

A further nursing specific questionnaire with 31 items was also generated. Following factor analysis, both questionnaires were shown to have internal consistency test and re-test and had high levels of validity and reliability (see Chapter 2).

The RPQ has been widely used and one example is its use in comparing role perceptions of nursing students in two nursing schools from two countries, in Portugal and Turkey (Sahin et al. 2013).

Attitudes to Health Professionals Questionnaire (AHPQ)

Lindqvist et al. (2005) reported a study devising a questionnaire to assess interprofessional attitudes. Using Kelly's construct theory as above, an exercise was undertaken with 20 members of staff initially across health schools in the University of East Anglia, UK. The 20 constructs generated were then tested on 190 students across a range of professions, medicine, nursing, midwifery, physiotherapy, nursing and occupational therapy. Each item was scored along a 10 cm visual analogue scale. Participants were asked ... 'where would you place a typical member of profession X on this scale'.

Examples included:

Caring   Not caring
Person centred   Technically focused

Analysis showed high internal consistency but variable test–retest reliability. The authors conclude that this 20-item questionnaire is a useful tool to assess interprofessional attitudes in health care settings.

The AHPQ was used to measure attitudes before and after a programme designed to encourage interdisciplinary pairs to have intentional conversations about clinical practice situations, be they positive or negative (Agarwal et al. 2008). The study involved two primary care teams affiliated to McMaster University, Hamilton, Ontario, Canada. Results showed increased knowledge and appreciation for others roles.

University of the West of England IP Questionnaire
Pollard et al. (2004) published a study describing the development of a questionnaire designed to measure attitudes and perceptions in regard to IP learning and working.

The study took place in the Faculty of Health and Social Care, University of the West of England (UWE), Bristol, UK. An expert faculty group generated a number of statements based on published work. Three scales were constructed:
1 Communication and teamwork ... students assess their communication and team skills.
2 Interprofessional learning scale ... exploring students attitudes to IP learning.
3 Interprofessional interaction scale ... exploring perceptions of interactions between professionals.

Each scale contains eight or nine statements that students rate along a Likert scale rating from 1 = strongly agree to 5 = strongly disagree. In the communications and teamwork scale two example statements are:

'I feel comfortable working in a group.'
'I feel uncomfortable taking the lead in a group.'

The authors describe three questionnaires, one at entry level, interim (second year) and final (nine months post qualification). The same questions are asked in each but in addition, demographic data are gathered at entry level.

There were a total of 643 respondents across health and social care professions including adult nursing, physiotherapy, social work, occupational therapy and radiotherapy.

The UWE Interprofessional Questionnaire has been used widely. In one example Ruebling et al. (2014) surveyed 350 students across nursing, nuclear medicine, physical therapy amongst others, in Saint Louis University St Louis, USA to compare attitudes before and after an introductory IPE experience.

Interprofessional Education Collaborative (IPEC) Assessment Tool

Dow et al. (2014) described a study with the aim of exploring the usefulness of the Interprofessional Education Collaborative (IPEC) competencies for assessing the effectiveness of IP education (see earlier in this chapter for more detail of these). The authors reviewed the 38 original IPEC competencies and adapted 32 as items. Five were further subdivided into 10 items and one competency was omitted as it referred to group as opposed to individual behaviour.

Items formed a question administered to a student population (n = 3236) in five health schools, Richmond, USA. Professions included were dentistry, medicine, pharmacy, allied health and nursing. There was a response of 481 (14.9%). Analysis defined four components that aligned to the original IPEC domains. The authors concluded that the IPEC competencies provide a useful tool for assessing the outcome of IP education.

A further iteration of this survey led to a shorter more user-friendly version of the tool consisting of two domains one linked to IP interaction and the other to IP values (Lockeman et al. 2016).

The following are validated team work instruments:

Team climate inventory

System for multiple level observations of groups

Team Climate Inventory (TCI)

Anderson and West (1998) described the development of a 5-factor 38-item questionnaire designed to measure different aspects of a team's collaborative processes. This was based on the four factor theory of climate for innovation in teams (West 1990), that is, those factors that predict innovation, which are:

Vision ... the vision is the higher level aim of the team with associated objectives that will help achievement of the aim. With clearly defined objectives the team's efforts become more focused.

Participative safety ... this refers to a climate where all are actively encouraged to contribute ideas in an environment that is perceived as supportive and non-threatening from a personal perspective.

Task orientation ... this refers to a generally high level of commitment in the team to excellence in task performance as evidenced by for example, a focus on individual and team accountability and control processes in place to monitor performance of the task.

Support for innovation ... this isn't just stated support for innovation but evidence of support in action in the behaviour of individuals in the team/ organisation.

The proposed items mapped to these factors were tested on a sample of 155 individuals from 27 hospital management teams and then on 971 individuals across 121 teams (35 primary care teams, 42 social services teams, 20 psychiatric teams and 24 oil company teams). Following factor analysis, five factors were identified, the original four and the additional – interaction frequency. This latter refers to the frequency of interaction within the team. This resulted in the 138-item Team Climate Inventory (TCI).

The TCI has been translated into a number of different languages and tested on a range of teams including, social services, primary care teams and management.

The application of TCI in a hospital-based setting in the Netherlands showed that it is a valid, reliable and discriminating self-report tool to measure team climate (Ouwens et al. 2008). In addition, a French version of the TCI has been validated for measuring Primary Care Teams processes (Beaulieu et al. 2014).

System for Multiple Level Observations of Groups (SYMLOG)

Bales and Cohen (1979) described the system for multiple observations of groups (SYMLOG) method for measuring interpersonal behaviour in teams. Bales developed the SYMLOG field theory based on observations of three bipolar dimensions in groups. These are:

Dominant vs submissive ... Teams that are characterised by dominance are likely to be outspoken, have high levels of participation whilst submissive teams are seen as passive.

Friendly vs unfriendly ... Friendly teams have high levels of co-operation and protectiveness of team members, that is, are very team centred as opposed to unfriendly teams that are individually centred. This has also been referred to as the level of sociability in the group.

Acceptance vs non-acceptance of task orientation of established authority ... This describes the team's acceptance of any rules and expectations of them.

Field theory assumes that these bipolar values can be located in a three dimensional space thus giving a visual representation of the current status of the team. These can be displayed as a bar diagram or field diagram.

The questionnaire comprises 26 statements of behaviour that the individual members of team rate from rarely, sometimes or often observed.

SYMLOG has been used to evaluate changes within a primary care team following interventions that included educational elements (Cashman et al. 2004).

Evaluation Frameworks/Models

Evaluation of learning and educational initiatives is vital. Any changes made to learners' experience need to be evaluated to ensure they are effective. In an educational setting in general, an educational initiative can be considered effective if:

1 it has on balance positive outcomes, for the individual, for the organisation, for patients/clients;
2 it is feasible, in terms of cost and the cost–benefit ratio;
3 it has no significant negative sequelae/side effects, or unintended negative effects.

There are a number of evaluation methods that are used widely across a number of sectors including education and some of them will be explored briefly.

Kirkpatrick's Four Level Model

When embarking on the evaluation of any learning it can be useful to follow Kirkpatrick's four-level model for assessing training effectiveness (Kirkpatrick 1994). The levels are:

- level 1 – *reaction* of the learner, how they felt about the experience, their initial reactions to a course, usually assessed through surveys, questionnaires or focus groups;
- level 2 – *learning*, this is a measure of the increase in knowledge that participants learned, usually assessed using criterion-referenced and before and after tests;
- level 3 – *behaviour*, this is change in behaviour in the workplace, transferring knowledge, skills and/or attitude from the learning environment to the workplace. It is recognised that it needs a certain period of time to convert learning into behaviour. This level is usually evaluated using observations and interviews with co-workers and supervisors;
- level 4 – *results*, this is the effect on the organisation or the wider environment as a result of the learning. This can be a measure of the financial impact of the course, that is, the return on investment.

There is still a misconception that with Kirkpatrick's levels that one starts in a sequential manner with level 1 and if resources and support allow build up to level 4. The correct way to use this approach is to start with level 4 and ask what result do we want/wish? Having said that Level 1 is perhaps still the most frequently used approach as it is the easiest to measure. Each level can however provide equally valuable information depending on the type of learning and type of leaners being evaluated.

There have been a number of modifications to Kirkpatrick's model based on criticisms that the model is too simplistic and that there is an implied causal relationship between each level that has not been tested.

Modifications include the Level 4 being split into two to reflect the impact on the organisation and the wider financial effects on the organisation and the wider community (Hamblin 1974). Kaufman et al. (1995) focused more on the wider societal value and Phillips (1995) on return on investment.

Specifically with in the field of IPE Barr et al. (2000), using Kirkpatrick's levels as a basis, revised the model to describe a sixfold typology for evaluating IPE.

Level 1 – 'reaction' is similar to Kirkpatrick's level 1 – this is the learners' views on the learning experience. There is however a difference with IPE learning experiences. There is with this a double responsibility. Level 1 is achieved if the learners remain positive and enthusiastic about learning with and about other professionals. The other side of the coin is that the experience should not be unsatisfactory, as there is a risk it could lead to the learners associating this negative experience with IP collaboration in real clinical settings.

Level 2a leads to changes in attitudes and perceptions whilst Level 2b leads to an increase in knowledge or skill. These have been separated out for practical purposes but it is important to remember that each is an essential element to effective learning in the IPE context.

Level 3 entails the learners transposing their level 2a and b positive changes into their clinical practice setting. With this level, there are it's own challenges since individual clinicians, in whatever profession, work in a complex system and the system needs to allow individuals the conditions to change their behaviour.

Level 4a leads to changes at the organisational level and level 4b where measurable benefits to patients /service users can be seen.

Barr's Dimensions

Harden's ladder has been described in Chapter 3. Another typology to reflect on is that of Barr (1996). In practice, the form of IPE will be determined by a range of issues, the aims of the programme, the engagement level of the learners and where the learning occurs. So in many ways any IPE learning can be a product of a number of trade-offs and negotiations. Barr's dimensions are described below and can be used as a useful checklist to benchmark any IPE.

Implicit or explicit
IPE can occur as a result of just bringing different professionals together.
   The unintended IPE. This can then be built upon and consolidated by more
   explicit learning such as workshops, short courses or programmes.
Discrete or integrated
The IPE can be a standalone learning experience or embedded within a wider
   programme in an integrated fashion.
All or part of a programme
In some circumstances, for example a postgraduate course, IPE may be the sole
   learning/teaching methodology. It is more common for the IPE to be just one
   element of a programme or course.
General or particular
IPE may focus on one particular learner group, in one specific setting or at the
   other end of the dimension it may have a broader application/use.
Positive or negative
As with any interaction, the IPE can have positive or negative results for the
   learners. This applies equally to trainers/faculty.
Individual or collective
The focus of IPE can be to meet one individual's learning needs or group /
   collective learning for small or larger teams.
Work/employment-based or college based
IPE can occur in the workplace, in the clinical setting in an informal or formal
   basis. Work place-based IPE tends to be task focused. In a university or college
   setting at undergraduate and postgraduate level the IPE will tend to be
   broader giving a more rounded experience.
Shorter or longer
At one end of the spectrum, IPE can be a very brief one off learning experience
   over a one-hour meeting. Generally the briefer the learning the more task-
   specific it is. At the other end of this dimension there are formal IP
   undergraduate programmes lasting years.
Early or later
The timing of the introduction of IPE in a professional career cycle is an important
   decision. It can be introduced from early days in an undergraduate programme,
   and then at various stages, immediately post qualification to on-going life- long
   learning.
Common or comparative content
Content can be shared or common across training programmes. This
   approach runs the risk of dilution of the professional identity. At the other
   extreme is specialist content and the bridge between these is comparative
   where different professions can compare roles and responsibilities and
   scope of practice.
Interactive or didactic
As discussed elsewhere in the book IPE to be successful relies on high levels of
   interaction between the professions involved. Therefore small group work is a
   common teaching strategy used, with either a case- or problem-based
   approach. Didactic approaches such as lectures tend to be used less often but
   may still have a part to play.

The InterProfessional Activity Classification Tool (InterPACT)

Xyrichis et al. (2017) described a review of published studies over the previous decade with the aim of exploring the use of terms related to IP activity/working. This was in part to attempt to validate a previously developed conceptual framework (Reeves et al. 2010).

They recognised the heterogeneity of IP definitions, educational interventions, participants and clinical areas examined without any conclusive results that can be easily reproduced and re-tested. The authors argue that there is a growing realisation that there is a requirement for a conceptual clarity as well as clarity in regard to definitions. The results of some studies have been accepted or endorsed by national quality agencies. The TeamSTEPPS intervention in North America has been endorsed by the Agency for Healthcare and Research and Quality (AHRQ) and in the UK the Multidisciplinary Team Feedback for Improving Teamwork (MDT-FIT) has been endorsed by the NHS Improving Quality (NHSIQ) (now subsumed into NHS England, (see Chapter 5 for more details on these two interventions and their impact).

Although these two examples are endorsed nationally in their own countries even these studies have contributed to the confusion surrounding terminology, and so on, conflating IP activity and team work.

Reeves et al. (2010) viewed IPP along six dimensions of the relationship of those working together;

Goals
Roles and responsibilities
Degree of shared identity
Commitment
Interdependence
Integration between clinical tasks

They matched these six different factors to four kinds of IP activity, teamwork, collaboration, co-ordination and networking. They provided descriptors of each of these.

Team work ... Encompasses a number of core elements including but not restricted to, a high level of shared team identity, clarity, interdependence, integration and shared responsibility. Examples of this type of interprofessional work can include family practice and emergency department/room teams.

Collaboration ... This is a looser form of interprofessional work. It differs from teamwork in that shared identity and integration of individuals are less important. However, it is similar to teamwork in requiring shared accountability and interdependence between individuals and clarity of roles/goals. Examples of this type of interprofessional work can be found across many general medical wards.

> *Co-ordination … This, as a form of IP work, is similar to collabora-*
> *tion in terms of shared identity. However, integration and interdepend-*
> *ence is less important. Co-ordination is similar to collaboration in that it*
> *does require some shared accountability between individuals and clarity*
> *of roles/tasks/goals. Examples of this type of IP work can be found in the*
> *case management literature which describes how individuals, usually*
> *called case managers co-ordinate the work of the other team members.*
>
> *Networking … A networking relationship is one in which shared team*
> *identity, clarity of roles/goals, interdependence, integration and shared*
> *responsibility are less essential. Networks can be virtual, in the sense that*
> *none of the members meet face to face, but communicate in an asynchro-*
> *nous manner via the internet, for example email or online conferencing).*
> *Examples of this type of IP work include networks of clinicians who meet*
> *to discuss or share information/clinical guidelines across a number of*
> *institutions.* (Reeves et al. 2010, p. 6)

In their follow up study 2017 following extensive review, Xyrichis et al. (2017) added two new sub-categories in the collaboration domain and three within the co-ordination one:

Collaboration	Consultative collaboration
	Collaborative partnership
Co-ordination	Co-ordinated collaboration
	Delegative co-ordination
	Consultative co-ordination

In terms of the six dimensions of IP activity, the authors offer definitions on each which are described as descriptors to guide researchers and clinicians.

Team commitment … This refers to the sense of attachment that the health care professionals feel towards their teams.

Team identity … This is the collection of meanings attached to their teams by the professionals.

Team goals … Explicit articulation of the purpose and aims of the team.

Team roles and responsibilities … This refers to the links between the professionals and their work … it's the extent to which a profession holds control over certain tasks.

Team interdependence … Is the extent to which an outcome of the IP interaction depends on decisions of all team members together.

Integration between work practices … This refers to how aligned the contribution of all professionals is to the desired outcome.

These definitions used as descriptors are a challenge. If one explores just one of these, team commitment, the authors state their descriptor is based on the work of Pearce and Herbik (2014). The latter reported a study of 71 change management teams in the car industry in the USA. The teams were surveyed exploring constructs that may affect team citizen behaviour (TCB). The latter is a complex construct itself made up of the following behaviours; altruism, civic virtue, consciousness, courtesy, team work and team mindedness. This concept of TCB derives from the work of George (e.g. George and Bettenhausen 1990) who focused on group as opposed to team factors that lead to success. In essence, the concept of team commitment as suggested by Xyrichis et al. (2017) is a complex one and it could be argued that without a clear operational definition just leads to more confusion.

The team work and networking as described in the 2010 paper remain as was. So they propose InterPACT as a tool /framework to classify types of IP work and interventions to promote or enhance IPE. The authors have described each kind of IP activity alongside six dimensions with levels of intensity from low/moderate/high and very high. The authors recognise that this is not the finished product but suggest that researchers into the effectiveness of IPE should use the framework to self-assess. That self-assessment they suggest involves two steps:

1 Reflection on the six dimensions: the reflection should focus on the judgement as to the extent to which each reflect the way of working.
2 Then discussion of this self-assessment alongside the four main types of IP activity, teamwork, collaboration, co-ordination or networking.

Each of the six activities are complex and although Xyrichis et al. (2017) state this as a basic model these can and will be open to broad and diverse interpretation.

This profile can then be described in the methodology of any protocol of evaluations into the effectiveness of IPE, hence, the authors argue, enabling a greater of ability to compare and contrast different studies. So in essence, this could be a practical tool to standardise practice and research in IPE and hence aid communication and understanding. It remains to be seen whether this argument will be realised.

Interprofessional Learning Outcomes

From the studies explored in Chapter 3, there are a number of key learning points. If the purpose of your study is to assess/evaluate the effective of IPE in a clinical setting follow the following rules:

1 Be clear about the professional profile of your participants.
2 Be clear about the numerical balance in each professional or discipline group.
3 Provide detailed demographics of your learners.

4 Describe your teaching method clearly. If small groups, describe how many over what period of time, how long? How many in each group, did profile vary over time, was there an attrition rate, if so was it greater for one profession compared to another?
5 Be clear about your aims, objectives, outcomes and curriculum.
6 Assess the learning process.
7 Assess the outcome for patients, individually or as groups.
8 Assess the impact on individual participants, knowledge, attitudes, behaviour.

Chapter Summary

There is a wide diversity of evaluation methods used in the published literature. This makes it a challenge to compare and contrast studies across the sector and difficult to replicate methodologies.

In this chapter the general principles of evaluation are explored including the elements of a project plan required to ensure a successful outcome. These include key steps such as the defining the scope, deciding on the research questions to be answered and the description of the methodology required to answer them. Practical issues such as data gathering, ethical considerations and data analysis are explored. A range of methods are widely used in data gathering including surveys, interviews and focus groups.

There is a wide range of specific assessment tools validated for use in the evaluation of IPE. These are described in detail along with two validated teamwork instruments.

Kirkpatrick's four step model of evaluation is described as well as the recently described InterPACT tool kit. The latter, may after testing provide a framework for researchers and educationalists to self-assess against to allow increased consistency and hence facilitate comparison and replicability of findings.

References

Adamson, J., Gooberman-Hill, R., Woolhead, G. et al. (2004). 'Questerviews': using questionnaires in qualitative interviews as a method of integrating qualitative and quantitative health services research. *Journal of Health Services Research & Policy* 9 (3): 139–145.

Agarwal, G., Idenouye, P., Hilts, L. et al. (2008). Development of a program for improving interprofessional relationships through intentional conversations in primary care. *Journal of Interprofessional Care* 22 (4): 432–435.

Anderson, N.R. and West, M.A. (1998). Measuring climate change for work group innovation: development and validation of the team climate inventory. *Journal of Organizational Behavior* 19: 235–258.

Babbie, E. (1973). *Survey Research Methods*. Belmont, CA: Wadsworth Publishing Company.

Bales, R.F. and Cohen, S.P. (1979). *SYMLOG: A Systematic Multiple Level Observation of Groups*. New York: Free Press.

Barceló, A., Cafiero, E., de Boer, M. et al. (2010). Using collaborative learning to improve diabetes care and outcomes: The VIDA project. *Primary Care Diabetes* 4 (3): 145–153.

Barr, H. (1996). Ends and means in interprofessional education; towards a typology. *Education and Health* 9 (3): 341–352.

Barr, H. and Brewer, M. (2012). Interprofessional practice-based education. In: Higgs, J., Barnett, R., Billett, S. et al. (Eds.) *Practice-Based Education. Practice, Education, Work and Society*, vol 6. Sense Publishers, Rotterdam. 119–212 doi: https://doi.org/10.1007/978-94-6209-128-3_15

Barr, H., Freeth, D., Hammick, M. et al. (2000). *Evaluations of Interprofessional Education: A UK Review for Health and Social Care*. CAIPE/BERA.

Barzansky, B. and Etzel, S.I. (2015). Medical schools in the United States. *Journal of the American Medical Association* 314 (22): 2426–2435.

Beaulieu, M.-D., Dragieva, N., Grande, C.D. et al. (2014). The team climate inventory as a measure of primary care teams' processes: validation of the French version. *Healthcare Policy* 9 (3): 40–54.

Berwick, D.M., Nolan, T.W., and Whittington, J. (2008). The triple aim: care, health and cost. *Health Affairs* 27: 759–769.

Boland, D., White, T., and Adams, E. (2018). Experiences of pharmacy trainees from an interprofessional immersion training. *Pharmacy* https://doi.org/10.3390/pharmacy6020037.

Bradburn, N., Sudman, S., and Wansink, B. (2004). *Asking Questions: The Definitive Guide to Questionnaire Design*. San Francisco: Jossey-Bass.

Cashman, S.B., Reidy, P., Cody, K. et al. (2004). Developing and measuring progress toward collaborative, integrated, interdisciplinary health care teams. *Journal of Interprofessional Education* 18 (2): 183–195.

Dillman, D. (2000). *Constructing the questionnaire*. Mail and internet surveys. New York: John Wiley & Sons.

Dow, A.W., DiazGranados, D., Mazmanian, P.E. et al. (2014). An exploratory study of an assessment tool derived from the competencies of the interprofessional education collaborative. *Journal of Interprofessional Care* 28 (4): 299–304.

Ekeh, P. (1974). *Social Exchange Theory: The Two Traditions*. Cambridge: Harvard University Press.

Gantt, H.L. (1910). *Work, wages and profit*. New York: Engineering Magazine; republished as Work, Wages and Profits. Easton, Pennsylvania: Hive Publishing Company. 1974.

Garfinkel, H. (1967). *Studies in Ethnomethodology*. Englewood Cliffs, NJ: Prentice-Hall.

George, J.M. and Bettenhausen, K. (1990). Understanding prosocial behavior, sales performance, and turnover. A group-level analysis in a service context. *Journal of Applied Psychology* 75: 698–709.

Glaser, B.G. and Strauss, A.L. (1967). *The Discovery of Grounded Theory: Strategies for Qualitative Research*. New York: Aldine de Gruyter.

Hamblin, A.C. (1974). *Evaluation and Control of Training*. New York: McGraw-Hill.

Hammersly, M. and Atkinson, P. (1983). *Ethnography: Principles in Practice*. London: Tavistock.

Hayward, K., Powell, L., and McRoberts, J. (1996). Changes in student perceptions of interdisciplinary practice in the rural setting. *Journal of Allied Health* 25 (4): 315–327.

Hind, M., Norman, I., Cooper, S. et al. (2003). Interprofessional perceptions of health care students. *Journal of Interprofessional Care* 17 (1): 21–34.

Horsburgh, M., Lamdin, R., and Williamson, E. (2001). Multiprofessional learning: the attitudes of medical, nursing and pharmacy students to shared learning. *Medical Education* 35: 876–883.

Iglesias, C. and Torgerson, D. (2000). Does length of questionnaire matter? A randomised trial of response rates to a mailed questionnaire. *Journal of Health Services & Research Policy* 5: 219–221.

Interprofessional Education Collaborative (2016). *Core Competencies for Interprofessional Collaborative Practice: 2016 Update*. Washington, DC: Interprofessional Education Collaborative.

Kaufman, R., Keller, J.M., and Watkins, R. (1995). What works and what doesn't: evaluation beyond Kirkpatrick. *Performance and Instruction* 35 (2): 8–12.

Kelly, G.A. (1955). *The Psychology of Personal Constructs*, vol. 1 and 2. New York: WW Norton.

Kirkpatrick, D.L. (1994). *Evaluating Training Programs: The Four Levels*. San Francisco: Berrett-Koehler.

Lindqvist, S., Duncan, A., Shepstone, L. et al. (2005). Development of the Attitudes to Health Professionals Questionnaire (AHPQ): a measure to assess interprofessional attitudes. *Journal of Interprofessional Care* 19 (3): 269–279.

Lockeman, K.S., Dow, A.W., DiazGranados, D. et al. (2016). Refinement of the IPEC competency self-assessment survey: results from a multi-institution study. *Journal of Interprofessional Care* 30 (6): 726–731.

Luecht, R., Madson, M., Taugher, M. et al. (1990). Assessing perceptions: design and validation of an interdisciplinary education perception scale. *Journal of Allied Health* 19: 181–191.

Mackay, S. (2004). The role perception questionnaire (RPQ): a tool for assessing undergraduate students' perceptions of the role of other professions. *Journal of Interprofessional Care* 18 (3): 289–302.

McFadyen, A.K., Webster, V., Strachan, K. et al. (2005). The readiness for interprofessional learning scale: a possible more stable sub-scale model for the original version of RIPLS. *Journal of Interprofessional Care* 19 (6): 595–603.

Norris, J., Carpenter, J.G., Eaton, J. et al. (2015). Development and construct validation of the interprofessional attitudes scale. *Academic Medicine* 90 (10): 1394–1400.

Ouwens, M., Hulscher, M., Akkermans, R. et al. (2008). The team climate inventory: application in hospital teams and methodological considerations. *Quality and Safety in Health Care* 17: 275–280.

Parsell, G. and Bligh, J. (1999). The development of a questionnaire to assess the readiness of health care students for interprofessional learning (RIRLS). *Medical Education* 33: 95–100.

Pearce, C.L. and Herbik, P.A. (2014). Citizenship behavior at the team level of analysis: the effects of team leadership, team commitment, perceived team support, and team size. *The Journal of Social Psychology* 144 (3): 293–310.

Phillips, J.J. (1995). Return on investment – Beyond the four levels. In E. F. Holton III (Ed.), *Academy of HRD 1995 Conference proceedings.*

Pollard, K.C., Miers, M.E., and Gilchrist, M. (2004). Collaborative learning for collaborative working? Initial findings from a longitudinal study of health and social care students. *Health and Social Care in the Community* 12 (4): 346–358.

Redline, C. and Dillman, D. (2002). The influence of alternative visual designs on respondents' performance with branching instructions in self-administered questionnaires. In: *Survey Nonresponse* (ed. R. Groves, D. Dillman, J. Eltinge, et al.), 179–194. New York: Wiley.

Reeves, S., Lewin, S., Espin, S. et al. (2010). *Interprofessional Teamwork for Health and Social Care.* Oxford, UK: Wiley-Blackwell.

Ruebling, I., Pole, D., Breitbach, A.P. et al. (2014). A comparison of student attitudes and perceptions before and after an introductory interprofessional education experience. *Journal of Interprofessional Care* 28 (1): 23–27.

Sahin, N.H., Tulek, Z., Rodrigues, M.A. (2013). The role perceptions of nursing students: A comparative study. 24th International Nursing Research Congress, Prague, Czech Republic 22–26 July 2013.

Smith, J.A. (2007). Hermeneutics, human sciences and health: linking theory and practice. *International Journal of Qualitative Studies on Health and Well-Being* 2: 3–11.

Thompson, R.S., Meyer, B.A., Smith-DiJulio, K. et al. (1998). A training program to improve domestic violence identification and management in primary care: preliminary results. *Violence and Victims* 13 (4): 395–410.

West, M.A. (1990). The social psychology of innovation in groups. In: *Innovation and Creativity at Work: Psychological and Organizational Strategies* (ed. M.A. West and J.L. Farr), 4–36. Chichester: Wiley.

Williams, B. and Webb, V. (2012). Examining the measurement properties of the Interdisciplinary Education Perception Scale (IEPS) in paramedic education. *Nurse Education Today* 33 (9): https://doi.org/10.1016/j.nedt.2012.10.015.

Xyrichis, A., Reeves, S., and Zwarenstein, M. (2017). Examining the nature of interprofessional practice: an initial framework validation and creation of the InterProfessional Acticvity Classification Tool (InterPACT). *Journal of Interprofessional Care* https://doi.org/10.1080/13561820.2017.1408576.

Zanotti, R., Sartor, G., and Canova, C. (2015). Effectiveness of interprofessional education by on-field training for medical students, with a pre-post design. *BMC Medical Education* https://doi.org/10.1186/s12909-015-0409-z.

Chapter 7 **The Future of Interprofessional Education**

What is the future of Interprofessional Education (IPE)? The history of IPE could be characterised by good times alternating with bad times.

Looking to the future there are fixed points for all health care systems in the world and the NHS in the UK is no exception. There are major challenges across the world in terms of the increasing need and demand from the population and the requirement to work differently, to move from a medical to a biosocial model. There is an imperative to move to a systems approach to health and social care workforce planning and development.

It is important to understand the definition of a system, which is a number of activities working to a common goal. It is recognised that the health system in it's current format and configuration is unsustainable.

Prudent Health Care

The principles of prudent heath care give a framework to allow conversations about change (Bradley and Wilson 2014). These principles are:

Do no harm. This is the principle that interventions which do harm or provide no clinical benefit are stopped;

Carry out the minimum appropriate intervention. The principle that treatment should begin with the basic proven tests and interventions. The intensity of testing and treatment is consistent with the seriousness of the illness and the patient's goals;

Organise the workforce around the 'only do what only you can do' principle. This is the principle that all clinical staff should operate at the top of their competence ceiling. For example, no-one should be seen by a General Practitioner when their needs could be met by an advanced paramedic.

How to Succeed at Interprofessional Education, First Edition. Peter Donnelly.
© 2019 John Wiley & Sons Ltd. Published 2019 by John Wiley & Sons Ltd.

Promote equity. This is the principle that what matters most is the individual patient's clinical needs.

The relationship between the user and the provider has to be reset to one of co-production.

The NHS

When looking ahead it is useful to reflect on the origins of the systems in which we work. The National Health Service (NHS) in the UK, upon which it is argued all other health systems are based, began in 1948. Aneurin Bevan, the then Health Secretary, launched the NHS at Park Hospital in Manchester (today known as Trafford General Hospital) on 5 July 1948. For the first time, hospitals, doctors, nurses, pharmacists, opticians and dentists were brought together under one umbrella organisation to provide services that were free for all at the point of delivery.

An extract from a leaflet sent to all households in February 1948 reads:

> **Your new National Health Service begins on 5th July. What is it? How do you get it?**
> *It will provide you with all medical, dental and nursing care. Everyone – rich or poor, man, woman or child-can use it or any part of it. There are no charges, except for a few special items. There are no insurance qualifications. But it is not a "charity". You are all paying for it, mainly as tax payers, and it will relieve your money worries in time of illness. (www.sochealth.co.uk/national-health-service/the-sma-and-the-foundation-of-the-national-health-service-dr-leslie-hilliard-1980/the-start-of-the-nhs-1948)*

The original concept implemented by Aneurin Bevan does not stand up to scrutiny across the UK. In England the current political climate has led, it could and has been argued, to the introduction of a level of market forces back into the delivery and planning of health care. Clinical commission groups (CCGs) were set up in England following the Health and Social Care Act 2012. The CCGs plan and commission health services for their geographical areas and are led by primary care staff with some secondary care input. CCGs are responsible for approximately two-thirds of the total NHS England budget of circ. £75 billion. Foundation Trusts in England are not-for-profit public benefit corporations that provide a significant percentage of all NHS hospital, mental health and ambulance services. The first wave of these were established in 2004 with many more coming on stream over the last few years.

In terms of population health the fixed points are:
1 the demographics of the population, living longer, multiple co-morbidity;
2 the challenges of over 50% of the population living with a chronic illness;
3 the increasing prevalence of dementia in all its forms as a function of just living longer; and
4 the emerging new cohorts of patients with complex unknown needs who are now survivors of major cancer.

The acceleration of the potential for technology to aid clinicians not just in education roles via high fidelity simulation but also the use of artificial intelligence in diagnostic procedures such as imaging.

Those in most need of good health and social care have least access to it. Julian Tudor Hart, a General Practitioner from Port Talbot, South Wales, first articulated this inverse care law (Hart 1971). He argued in his original paper that this was due to a range of social inequalities. These health inequalities continue today. The strategic review of health inequalities in England (Marmot et al. 2010) highlighted the impact of social gradient on health outcomes, the avoidable differences in health outcomes. The review called for action to reduce the gradient in health by tackling those social determinants of health that have the most impact.

We are now in the third medical revolution. The first was the public health revolution epitomised by the discovery that the 1854 cholera outbreak in London was as a result of contaminated water via the water pump on Broad Street, in the Soho area (now Broadwick Street), and not air borne. This finding led to the emergence of public health medicine.

The second has been the technological revolution over the last 50 years with investment in evidence based medicine and quality focus, for example Magnetic Resonance Imaging, coronary artery bypass graft surgery, joint replacements, chemotherapy, renal dialysis, to mention just a few.

The Third Medical Revolution

We are now at the beginning of the third medical revolution which is being driven by mobile technology, specifically the smart phone. This is driving a revolution putting citizens in control of their own data, increasing their knowledge. An example is the smart phones that allow patients to self-monitor their blood pressure, blood glucose, and electrocardiograph and hence have control. This allows patient access to diagnostics and monitoring, facilitating self-management. Some of these have been approved by the United States Food and Drugs Administration Agency (FDA). This will allow the sea change of individual citizens having ownership of their own data moving to semi-autonomous individualised medicine (Topol 2016).

For Patient-centred care (PCC) to succeed there are some requirements.

The first is 'activated patients' who are active participants in their own health care. Activated patient behaviours include:

Taking responsibility for one's own health care needs;

Diagnosing and self-managing minor ailments;

Working in partnership with health care professionals to choose the most appropriate treatment; and

Actively managing any long-term condition.

The PCC is a part of a larger movement that is redefining the relationship between the citizen and the health system. The requirement for this re-alignment/recalibration is the changed demographic of service users, financial constraints and medical technology.

Patient activation has been shown to depend on a number of factors, levels of knowledge, skill and confidence and as these are competencies they can be learnt (Hibbard and Gilburt 2014).

> *Every patient is an expert in their chosen field, namely themselves and their own life.* (Hill 2014)

One example where the engaged or activated patient is central is the 'House of Care Model' (Coulter et al. 2013). This is a systems approach with person-centred care at the heart. The walls are the activated patient and a workforce that are engaged actively with collaborative working, who are in that IPE space. These two pillars form the walls of the House of Care. Overarching these is the organisational commitment to the person-centred approach and underpinning these is workforce planning with a multiprofessional systems approach.

Patient activation can be measured using the patient activation measure (PAM) that comprises 13 statements covering beliefs, confidence and management of health tasks and self-assessed knowledge (Mukoro 2012). Analyses of PAM gives four levels of patient activation from passive at one extreme to adoption of most of the behaviours needed to support self-management.

Patient activation in IPE could act as key lever for systems change, behavioural change across the education and training and health and social care sector. So building in the need /evidence of the effectiveness and value of patients for MP team work across agencies into any patient or citizen activation programmes is likely to help enhance IPE.

The innovations taking place at a range of undergraduate and postgraduate and NHS organisations are echoed in many other colleges and universities around the world. There is much support and optimism that real collaborative learning experiences can and will transfer to the future practice of these students after they graduate and move on to their professional careers.

There is clearly an argument that efforts to achieve collaborative practice by introducing IPE were not always successful because education/training and clinical practice were not as closely aligned as they should be.

What Has Held IPE Back?

The multitude of terms with differing definitions as described in Chapter 3 and the resultant confusion have acted as barriers to IPE progress globally (Xyrichis et al. 2017).

Pre-conceived ideas of one professional group in regard to others can act as a barrier to successfully integrating IPP. The argument is that early exposure to IPE (Ateah et al. 2011) can help improve perception of other professions and facilitate the breakdown in stereotypes.

Clark (2011) reflects on the seven deadly sins, of organising and developing IPE, a metaphor that reflects the barriers to the promotion of IPE. As one example he defined lust as:

> the obsessive attraction to one's own profession, a kind of academic auto-eroticism. (Clark 2011, p. 322)

So, this inward-looking obsession of most professions, perpetuated on occasions by the fundamental structures in universities with essentially uniprofessional health schools for example, leads to a major barrier to the promotion of IPE.

Lessons from successes of the enhancement and adoption of IPE such as in Curtin University and the Nexus (see Chapter 6) have been described. These include ensuring engagement of the learners, the faculty, the institution and external partners. Barnsteiner et al. (2007) summarised these into six criteria for full engagement in IPE namely;

1 That IPE is embedded in the fabric of the organisation and is well known, accepted, observable and measurable. That it is explicit.

2 That faculty from different professional backgrounds co-create the learning experiences. Not one profession dominates. That it is true co-production.

3 Learners have planned and opportunistic opportunities built into their learning schedule to experience and rehearse collaborative practice, team working and how these processes link to improved patient experience and the value patients place on these.

4 IPE is explicitly embedded in the curriculum and learners are aware that it is a requirement.

5 Learners are assessed mapped to agreed IPE competencies.
6 Organisational/institutional infrastructure supports faculty to develop and enhance the IPE experience.

Developments in IPE in the Last 20 Years

The increasing interest in IPE has been reflected in the activity across the globe and manifested in an increasing volume and quality of published work. There is a wide range of novel approaches to the design, delivery and assessment of IPE-like activity. However, there remain barriers for the conditions to allow IPE to have the recognition/importance it needs and deserves.

These barriers include:

1 the type of studies published, small numbers, single sites;
2 the lack of the use of theory in IPE work;
3 the use of the various terms as described in Chapter 2 varies considerably which does not allow comparisons and replication of studies;
4 a lack of clarity in regard to leadership roles for IPE;
5 a lack of evidence for impact on the triple aim (quadruple aim); and
6 a lack of learner-led IPE initiatives.

What Are the Keys to Unlock the Potential of IPE?

Leadership in IPE

There is a recognised need to move from a traditional service-delivery model to one that is patient-outcome driven. A single system of seamless care for health and social care in any country can only be delivered if four specific aims are met, the quadruple aim (Bohenheimer and Sinsky 2014):

1 Improve population health and wellbeing through a focus on prevention.
2 Improve the experience and quality of care for individuals and families.
3 Enrich the wellbeing, capability and engagement of the health and social care workforce.
4 Increase the value achieved from funding of health and care through improvement, innovation, use of best practice, and eliminating waste.

This approach of an outcome-based health care system brings into the focus the collaboration that is needed to deliver IP care (McCallin 2003).

The IP approach to the delivery of care is team based, with a shared jointly owned set of aims leading to shared responsibility without the traditional hierarchy. For this to be achieved there needs to be a changing approach to leadership. There is still the assumption that the traditional leadership model is applicable in health and social care. This doesn't take fully into account the complexities of clinical care, with patients at their most vulnerable, so there is a requirement for specialised collaborative care, delivered by teams comprising different professionals and different disciplines within those professions. So, the key to high quality services is skilled IP team leaders who can drive innovative models of care.

In IP leadership all team members carry a level of responsibility for team processes and hence team outcomes, that is outcomes for patients. Implicit in this is the need for all team members to actively take on informal and formal (with the title) leadership roles. These roles will shift and flex depending on the clinical needs of the patients at any given point. There is an intrinsic fluidity in this approach. This is about equal responsibility and equal participation of all professions driven by the needs of the patients. That is the theory that is to a large part based on the premise that all health and social care professional will change the way they think in practice.

This shared leadership may be easier to realise in smaller more fixed, established teams that do not have a rapid turnover. Also, before responsibility for leadership can be shared individuals have to earn that privilege, that is they have to display competency in the role to colleagues.

Another concept worth exploring further is that of stewardship as an underlying philosophy for IP teams. (Block 1996) defines it as:

accountability without control or compliance.

Stewardship maintains accountability for control but importantly doesn't centralise or place leadership with one individual. It is about the concept of looking after the system, not owning it.

So how practical is this shared leadership for the future of IPE? Reeves et al. (2010) reflect on some of the barriers to this approach. The concept of medical dominance over other health and social care professionals is one issue described in detail by Turner (1995). The perception of medical dominance remains an ongoing issue. The flexibility in leadership roles, as patients follow a care pathway, is a challenge for individual practitioners and the team itself. There is as yet, little or no support for the development of skills in this area. For the future, this is required. A lever or catalyst for this is the increasing focus on patient-centred care including the need for further alignment between education and clinical governance within heath-care organisations. This should mean that all staff members have specific development opportunities mapped to their leadership roles in IP teams and recognised explicitly in their scope of practice. Through the 1990s there emerged the notion of the organisational 'hero' (The Kings Fund 2011). There was, however, recognition that organisations could not rely on a model of the charismatic leader and there emerged a move towards more distributed or collaborative approaches (Fullan 2001). This shared leadership model it is argued gained traction in the NHS as a result of the emergence of the multidisciplinary team as pivotal, in clinical terms, to the successful delivery of services. It is argued that leadership is not confined to a small number of individuals as a consequence of their position in a hierarchical organisation but that all members can and should have a leadership role (Pearce and Conger 2003).

This has been further elaborated on by Ancona and Bresman (2007) who describe X teams. X teams engage in high levels of external activity combined with extreme execution inside the team with the flexibility to change core tasks. The authors argued that good teams frequently failed as they are too inward looking. Central to this model is distributed leadership.

The issue of leadership for IP practice has received more attention in the last five years with more published in the literature. Brewer et al. (2016) summarise a number of leadership approaches in the NHS:

1 Collective;
2 Transformational (distributed);
3 Network theory (Baker et al. 2010);
4 Quantum leadership (Montgomery 2011); and
5 Dynamic delegation (Dow et al. 2017).

Despite these examples there is little published work describing theories of IP leadership and this is clearly an area that will require further attention.

Montgomery's quantum leadership (2011) describes an innovative education programme for Doctorates of nursing leaders based on complex adaptive systems and quantum leadership theories (Porter-O'Grady and Mulloch 2011). Quantum leadership has its origins in complexity theory and chaos theory and can be summarised in 10 principles:

Wholes are made up of parts.

All health care is local.

Adding value to a part adds value to the whole.

Complex systems are made up of simple systems.

Diversity is a necessity of life.

Error is essential to creation.

Systems thrive when all of their functions intersect and interact.

Equilibrium and disequilibrium are in constant tension.

Change is generated from the centre outward.

Revolution results from the aggregation of local changes.

The quantum theory of leadership describes that team players do their share of work and hold others in the team accountable for the expected outcomes. This plays into the other views of leadership around joint accountability.

Going forward there is a need to align IPE and the needs and requirements of the NHS. There is a growing recognition of the need to place patient values at the core of care provision. Putting the patient at the centre requires a change in culture and, hence to achieve this, a change in behaviour.

The concept of compassionate leadership has been shown to lead to improvements in patient outcomes but these are not achieved in isolation. One wall of the House of Care is the activated patient. So, to enhance IPE/IPPP engagement with patients/citizens is essential. Strategies such as training to enhance citizens' knowledge, skills and confidence in health and social care choices are essential.

The elements of compassionate care are (West et al. 2017):

1 Paying attention … active listening so that as a leader one can identify the challenges that staff are facing. Attending to these challenges can allow in-depth exploration, which leads to greater understanding. This active listening should be without judgement and without apportioning or seeking to apportion blame.

2 Taking steps to understand the position the staff, groups of staff, are in is important. The more staff are encouraged to have a deeper understanding of their challenges the more likely they are to be empowered to make the changes required. An element of this is using coaching behaviours to help others discover their own solutions.

3 Empathising increases team members' motivation, drive and engagement. Empathy also generates a more positive emotional working environment facilitating creativity (novel solutions) and innovation (adapting ideas from elsewhere to meet the business needs of the organisation).

4 Taking thoughtful and intelligent action is the fourth element of compassionate leadership. This can allow team members to evaluate different options in a safe environment.

The health and social care systems are adaptive complex systems. There is growing evidence that there is a requirement for specific leadership skills in this arena. The characteristics of a system leader include (Fillingham and Weir 2014):

Ability to work across organisations and across sectors, multiple systems;
Ability to cope with ambiguous issues, uncertainty, complexity;
Working collaboratively across traditional boundaries;
Ability to co-create a shared vision; and
Being curious, attentive, externally facing with a coaching capability.

These emerging requirements of health and social care systems' leaders mirror those of IPE leaders providing the conditions for IPE to be enhanced for the benefit of citizens.

There is a wider issue with IPE. As healthcare educators, we have to be acutely aware of the changing working environment of health care learners

(Thistlethwaite 2016). These two worlds have for too long been disjoined or at best, the education space lags behind developments in the NHS.

At the same time the NHS and other health care systems are under extreme pressure, winter pressures, generally increased demand, shortages in specialties and shortages in professions. These pressures act as levers for innovation and creativity further misaligning health education from the service.

In addition, there is limited evidence in published IP studies for a significant impact on the triple aim. In a review of the literature, Brandt et al. (2014) found limited reference to the triple aim in work over a 40-year period.

There is a need for exposure to IP practice early in health careers in order to normalise this. Examples are longitudinal integrated clerkships and student-led (in medicine) clinics.

Thistlethwaite raises the concept of whether there is such a thing as an interprofessional identity similar to the professional identity. She argues that perhaps it is best to think of this concept in the terms of … becoming an interprofessional. More work is needed in this area to unravel the factors that contribute to an evolving construct of the self as an interprofessional.

Baker et al. (2010) described a network model for faculty development. Although the model described is located in a medical school it is applicable across professions. Based on network theory the authors offer a conceptualisation of a faculty development model based on seven inter linked factors, the fishhook model that supports development.

Team Work – A Redundant Term?

Despite progress in the recognition of the importance of IP practice there is still limited evidence of high-impact, reproducible interventions that are shown to improve team working (a common concept) that then lead to better health outcomes for patients. Dow et al. (2017) explored the teams involved in providing care for 100 patients with colorectal cancer. They described a range of complex networks of health care professionals, some small numbers, others larger, some with loose associations, others with close day-to-day collaboration. There the concept of 'the team' does not really apply. In addition, it is a challenge to design educational interventions for these heterogeneous networks. In addition, these networks evolve in terms of associations, consistent members and professions. That is, they are not static. So the traditional model of educational interventions for teams such as:

1 Define what the team does.
2 Design interventions to help the team deliver these.
3 Train the team tighter.
4 Use feedback to drive further training.

These broad principles are a challenge to apply to fluid networks. The authors suggest different levels of network competencies (NCs), first generalised NCs for all, for example, to understand how information about patients flows through complex health systems. As electronic patient records become more ubiquitous and sophisticated, competencies in networking within that 'virtual' electronic space will be increasingly important. Then more focused enhanced NCs for what they describe as central health case staff – those with increased responsibility.

The driver for more widespread adoption of IPE and IPP has to be patient need. The health care needs of the population, at whatever point individual patients (and their relatives) are on the care pathway, are delivered best by each profession working collaboratively in a team. To work in any team your performance will be enhanced if you understand the roles and responsibilities and constraints/limitations of team members around you.

Chapter 3 explored the evidence for the effectiveness of IPE and related learning activities. The evidence from these studies is at best ambiguous. Further clarity is need.

How do we ensure that IPE for health professions' education will have influence on collaborative practice in the real world. What about the lingering resistance to collaborative education and practice? How do we break down the remaining silos that exist in both arenas? The answer is evidence. Evidence to support the enhanced roll out of IPE to support and maximise the activities of MDTs (MPTs), in an integrated fashion, to ensure patients have the best service to meet their health and social needs.

The Role of Health and Social Care Regulators

Is there an opportunity to set the conditions whereby different health regulators approve or accredit joint areas/ scopes of work such as IP practice?

In the UK the nine regulatory bodies set the educational requirements needed to enter a profession and the standards required to practice safely and effectively. In the UK there was a consultation on the role of health and social care regulators in 2018. There is a view that the number of health and social care regulators leads to confusing and inconsistent educational requirements. One proposal suggested in the consultation, is that by merging regulators there is scope for a new and consistent single approach to, and harmonisation of, standards and the approach to education across the professions. Although this only at present applies to the UK the principles outlined could be applied globally. So if there is a drive towards joint regulation that facilitates joint accreditation of areas of work, or scopes of practice, one such area should be IP practice as part of the professional development required to gain that accreditation.

Practical Tools

One essential requirement is a simple practical tool that educators can use to check against so that published work can be accurately compared. Such a tool could emerge from the framework described by Xyrichis et al. (2017). What is required is a very practical tool that can be used to allow a clear description and understanding of the IPE elements and the level/extent of IPE activity. Without this, as can be seen in some of the published work, any statistically significant changes as a result of the IPE may be as a result of generic, non-specific effects of the educational experience and /or unplanned networking, the hidden IPE curriculum.

Reflective Portfolios

Domac et al. (2016) describe a study in Leicester exploring the use of reflective portfolios by social work students to assess their value in promoting IP learning. Portfolios are widely used across the health and social care sector as an assessment tool to facilitate life-long learning. Different elements are used in the portfolio including case discussion, with the aim of helping the individuals to develop critical thinking and reflection. The study reported that although the social work students found reflective writing a challenge the portfolio as a tool was perceived as an effective way to increase their ability to reflect in an interprofessional setting. So, it could be argued that further work is needed to see what elements of portfolio work could help this.

The whole issue of health and social care practitioners feeling safe in a portfolio space has been highlighted by the Dr. Bawa-Garba case (Godlee 2018). There have been fears not just within the medical profession in regard to how reflections in portfolios may be used by the courts in criminal or other cases.

From an educational point of view, there are concerns about the possible unintended consequences for learning and reflective practice not just for trainee doctors through their respective postgraduate specialty ePortfolios, which are required for progression, but also for all health professionals who are required to reflect as a key process within their annual appraisal and hence revalidation or licencing.

Student Lead IPE

As a result of the change in funding models for university education and the changing expectation of the millennials, there has been a sea change in education at all levels. Within Higher Education Institutions students are increasingly co-creators of knowledge and the learners as partners in education development is important.

Students at one end of the continuum are involved in designing and leading learning and at the other end students themselves initiate the learning. There is a need for peer-to-peer and co-peer IPE activity.

Virtual Communities

In the area of digitalisation, virtual learning environments have been with us for some period of time. As discussed in Chapter 4, Walsh and van Soeren (2012) consider the use of technology to aid the delivery and dissemination of IPE as the future direction of travel for all learning and IPE in particular. A review of the use of virtual communities of practice to improve IP collaboration (McLoughlin et al. 2018) highlights the range of opportunities for virtual communities of practice that can facilitate informal support for IPP particularly reducing social and professional isolation. In addition the third medical revolution (the health revolution that we are in) will lead to citizens having and owning their own data digitally and as a result being more informed and more able to participate in shared decision making. There needs to be the strategic, political and value-based links made between new models of care and the role that IPE can play in acting as a catalyst, an enabler, for change and a factor in a new sustainable paradigm.

For a truly patient-centred care model all health and social care professionals need to work in a collaborative way and they can only undertake that role if they each understand the roles and responsibilities and scope of practice of all other professionals in that care pathway. IPE is the golden thread that runs through all of these pathways.

Chapter Summary

So are we asking the wrong question when we ask … does IPE work? Perhaps, what we should ask is: how effective is an MDT or rather an MPT in improving patient outcomes and enhancing the experience of patients?

The history of IPE is chequered, with many ups and an equal number of downs. There are strategic frameworks that can help this agenda including prudent health care principles.

We are now in the third medical revolution driven by patients, knowledge and mobile technology, the smart phone. What is the future role of IPE in this revolution? The answer lies in the principles of patient-centred care, driven by the patient.

Barriers to IPE are well rehearsed and solutions will require leadership in IPE, systems leadership skills. One such model is compassionate leadership that has been shown to improve patient outcomes. There are challenges to team working offered, with the argument made for the greater importance of networks. How will IPE play into this agenda?

There is a need for practical tools so that a greater level of evidence and consistency of IPE evaluations can tease out which specific elements are most effective. There is the additional need for learners to be genuinely involved in the co-creation of their own IPE with the innovative use of virtual communities.

The triple and quadruple aims are the standards that are applied to any health and social care service. These should be a focus for researchers and educationalists exploring the impact of IPE.

So, although the story of IPE is actually an old one, it has opened a new chapter in health professions' education. Nurses and other healthcare professionals who are thinking about going back to school will find that the disciplines are not as isolated as they once seemed to be, and healthcare education has closer ties to practice than ever before.

References

Ancona, D. and Bresman, H. (2007). *X-teams: How to Build Teams that Lead, Innovate and Succeed*. Boston, MA: Harvard Business Review Press.

Ateah, C.A., Snow, W., Wener, P. et al. (2011). Stereotyping as a barrier to collaboration: does interprofessional education make a difference? *Nurse Education Today* 31: 208–213.

Baker, l., Reeves, S., Egan-Lee, E. et al. (2010). The ties that bind: a network approach to creating a programme in faculty development. *Medical Education* 44: 132–139.

Barnsteiner, J.H., Disch, J.M., Hall, l. et al. (2007). Promoting interprofessional education. *Nursing Outlook* 55: 144–150.

Block, P. (1996). *Stewardship*. San Francisco: Berrett-Koehler.

Bohenheimer, T. and Sinsky, C. (2014). From triple to quadruple aim: care of the patient requires care of the provider. *Annals of Family Medicine* 12 (6): 573–576.

Bradley, P. and Wilson, A. (2014). *Achieving Prudent Healthcare in NHS Wales*. Cardiff: Public Health Wales http://www.1000livesplus.wales.nhs.uk/sitesplus/documents/1011/Achieving%20prudent%20healthcare%20in%20NHS%20Wales%20paper%20Revised%20version%20%28FINAL%29.pdf (accessed: 30 June 2018).

Brandt, B., Lutfiyya, M.N., King, J.A. et al. (2014). A scoping review of interprofessional collaborative practice and education using the lens of the Triple Aim. *Journal of Interprofessional Education* 28 (5): 393–399.

Brewer, M.L., Flavell, H.L., Trede, F. et al. (2016). A scoping review to understand 'leadership' in interprofessional education and practice. *Journal of Interprofessional Care* 30 (4): 408–415.

Clark, P.G. (2011). The devil is in the details: the seven deadly sins of organizing and continuing interprofessional education in the US. *Journal of Interprofessional Care* 25: 321–327.

Coulter, A., Roberts, S., and Dixon, A. (2013). *Delivering Better Services for People with Long-term Conditions. Building the House of Care*. London: The Kings Fund.

Domac, S., Anderson, E.S., and Smith, R. (2016). Learning to be interprofessional through the use of reflective portfolios? *Social Work Education* 35 (5): 530–546.

Dow, A.W., Zhu, X., Sewell, D. et al. (2017). Teamwork on the rocks: rethinking interprofessioanl practice as networking. *Journal of Interprofessional Care* 31 (6): 677–678.

Fillingham, D. and Weir, B. (2014). *System Leadership; Lessons and Learning from AQuA's Integrated Care Discovery Communities* (ed. London). The King's Fund.

Fullan, M. (2001). *The New Meaning of Educational Change*, 3e. London: Routledge Falmer.

Godlee, F. (2018). There but for the grace of God. *The British Medical Journal* 360: k485.

Hart, J.T. (1971). The inverse care law. *The Lancet* 297: 405–412.

Hibbard, J. and Gilburt, H. (2014). *Supporting People to Manage Their Health: An Introduction to Patient Activation*. London: Kings Fund www.kingsfund.org.uk/sites/default/files/field/field_publication_file/supporting-people-manage-health-patient-activation-may14.pdf (accessed: 30 June 2018).

Hill, E. (2014). Smart patients. *The Lancet* 15: 140–141.

Marmot, M.G., Allen, J., Goldblatt, P. et al. (2010). *Fair Society: Healthy Lives: Strategic Review of Health Inequalities in England Post-2010*. London UK: The Marmot Review.

McCallin, A. (2003). Interdisciplinary team leadership: a revisionist approach for an old problem. *Journal of Nursing Management* 11: 364–370.

McLoughlin, C., Patel, K.D., O'Callaghan, T. et al. (2018). The use of virtual communities of practice to improve interprofessional collaboration and education: findings from an integrated review. *Journal of Interprofessional Care* 32 (2): 136–142.

Montgomery, K.L. (2011). Leadership redefined: educating the doctorate of nursing practice nurse leaders through innovation. *Nursing Administration Quarterly* 35: 248–251.

Mukoro, F. (2012). Summary of the Evidence on performance of the patient Activation measure (PAM). http://personcentredcare.health.org.uk/sites/default/files/resources/patientactivation-1.pdf (accessed: 30 September 2018).

Pearce, C.L. and Conger, J.A. (2003). All those years ago: the historical underpinnings of shared leadership. In: *Shared Leadership: Reframing the Hows and Whys of Leadership* (ed. C.L. Pearce and J.A. Conger), 1–18. Thousand oaks, CA: Sage.

Porter-O'Grady, T. and Mulloch, K. (2011). *Quantum Leadership: Advancing Innovation, Transforming Health Care*, 3e. Sudbury, MA: Jones & Barlett Learning.

Reeves, S., MacMillan, K., and Van Soeren, M. (2010). Leadership of interprofessional health and social care teams: a socio-historical analysis. *Journal of Nursing Management* 18: 258–264.

The King's Fund, (2011). The future of leadership and management in the NHS. No more heroes. Report from The King's Fund Commission on Leadership and Management in the NHS. https://www.kingsfund.org.uk/sites/default/files/future-of-leadership-and-management-nhs-may-2011-kings-fund.pdf (accessed 30 September 2018).

Thistlethwaite, J. (2016). Interprofessional education: 50 years and counting. *Medical Education* 50 (11): 1082–1086.

Topol, E. (2016). *The Patient Will See You Now: The Future of Medicine is in Your Hands*. New York: Basic Books.

Turner, B.S. (1995). *Medical Power and Social Knowledge*. London: Sage.

Walsh, M. and van Soeren, M. (2012). Interprofessional learning and virtual communities: an opportunity for the future. *Journal of Interprofessional Care* 26: 43–48.

West, M., Eckert, R., Collins, B. et al. (2017). *Caring to Change. How Compassionate Leadership Can Stimulate Innovation in Health Care*. London: The Kings Fund.

Xyrichis, A., Reeves, S., and Zwarenstein, M. (2017). Examining the nature of interprofessional practice: an initial framework validation and creation of the InterProfessional Acticvity Classification Tool (InterPACT). *Journal of Interprofessional Care* https://doi.org/10.1080/13561820.2017.1408576.

Index

How to Succeed at Interprofessional Education, First Edition. Peter Donnelly.
© 2019 John Wiley & Sons Ltd. Published 2019 by John Wiley & Sons Ltd.

158 **Index**